EASY GUIDE TO
Mesmerism & Hypnotism

An exposition of the secrets of mesmerism,
clairvoyance, hypnotism, will-force
and mind-reading

J. Coates, Ph.D.

TABLE OF CONTENTS

INTRODUCTION.

This work dealing with the science of Mesmerism is written by J, Coates, P.H.D., who says as follows—it is written in everyday language, and may limp a little here and there. For none of these faults do I offer an apology to my readers. I ask them to take it as it is—as something more than a mere introduction to a most interesting and important subject.

My personal relation to the greatest and most successful Mesmerists of the day—both in private and public life—Captain Hudson, Dr. Spencer T. Hall, Captain John James, Dr. William Hitchman; the friends and contemporaries of Drs. Elliotson, Braid, and Gregory; Harriet J. Martineau, H. G. Atkinson, F. G. S., and others—has not been without a marked —shall I say "Mesmeric"—influence on myself, contributing in no mean degree to my acquaintance with the subject, experience, and well known career as a public Mesmerist.

Dr. Roth, President of the British Homoeopathic Society, admits the facts of Mesmerism, and contributes learned articles on the subject to the Society and its journal. He declares: "we cannot any longer afford to sneer at the miracles performed at the institution, known by the name of Bethshan, since we have healers in our midst who dispense with both *physic* and *faith*. These healers are medical men." These are important contributions and admissions. They will have some influence with the public, who are always more or less influenced by the opinions of the Faculty.

Medical men have a weakness for experiment. I should very much regret to see the sneer and abuses arising from the mal-administration of Mesmerism and Hypnotism, which are now and have been besetting Continental hospital practice, extending to this country.

Experimenting with hysterical and diseased patients is at once to be deprecated in the strongest possible language. Experiments should not be indulged which are not essentially curative and normally elevating in character. *This is not done*, I am sorry to say. The gratification of idle and pedantic curiosity, in the operations of these modem Hypnotists, appears to me to be the predominating motive, the CURATIVE, being left to the *accidental provings*.

I look to the honour and common sense of the Faculty as a whole to put down any such attempts here. I rejoice to note the fact that much of the continental practice is impossible here, owing to the stamina or difference in the constitutions and mental capacity of the people at home compared with those abroad.

The following extract from the Paris letter of *The British Medical Journal*, January 1, 1887, will be interesting to read in connection with the foregoing structures: —

Mr. Jules Voisin has made two highly interesting experiments, at Salpetriere Hospital, on hysterical patients on whom he studied the action of telepathic remedies (*medicamentia distance*), such as metals and the magnet. He explained the phenomenon of various changes of personality presented by one of his patients, M. V. the same individual who was experimented on by MM. Bourru and Butot (See *Congress of Grenoble*, 1885, and *Societe de Biolegic*, 1885). M. Voisin's experiments Were made with corked and sealed phials of an opaque colour. He was himself ignorant of the contents of these phials, and was careful not to utter a word in the patient's presence. He threw the subject into a lethargic, somnolent and cataleptic state, but obtained no result under these conditions. When M. Voisin made his experiments on any patient in a waking state, the latter immediately fell into a *hypnotic state, and exhibited symptoms of disturbance, nausea and vomiting.* If the name of a drug, of which the effects are well known, or the effects of any medicament whatsoever were mentioned, during the state of hypnotism, the patient immediately manifested the physiological effects of these remedies. *Suggestion and unconscious suggestion were thus manifested.* In another series of experiments, M. Jules Voisin observed during one of the three phases of somnolence (lethargy, somnambulism, catalepsy), the state of one of his subjects Y.; he was not affected by the magnet. In the walking state no effect took place unless the magnet was seen by the patient, when it induced and attacked probably through suggestion. *Gold and mercury caused redness and blisters* if V. was aware of their presence; these results were obtained likewise during somnambulism. By suggestion, the effect of metals was destroyed or produced without their presence, and if the contract of metal took place without the knowledge of V. when he was awake, no effect occurred. *General sensibility, sensory and motor sensibility and the psychical state were effected by suggestion.* M. Jules Voisin therefore believes it possible that the phenomenon of change of personality, as described by MM. Bourru and Butot, represents the *last phase of a hysterical attack, a phase characterized by delirium with delusions, and lasting several months.* Similar changes of personality, lasting only a short time, were observed in Somnambulism. They were always preceded by a physical change resembling an attack, and they were apparently induced, by any mental suggestion which accidentally recalled the previous existence of V. — [*The italics are mine.*]

The whole of these experiments are for the purpose of supporting. "The Theory of Suggestion—or Hypnotism" as opposed to the Theory of Mesmerism or Animal Magnetism. In the following pages the difference between Animal Magnetism and Hypnotism, may be traced throughout every chapter. Belonging to the old school of Mesmerists, I have a weakness for Animal Magnetism as the primary operating agent in all mesmeric phenomena. At the same time, I have always known and recognised the influence of other agents or secondary causes, such as *weariness of flesh and spirit, suggestion and imagination*, made so much of now-a-days by hypnotists.

These powers then, which medical men and others are beginning to realise can be exercised effectively, and with good and evil results, should as far as possible be kept out of the hands of inexperienced novices and unscrupulous operators. Whether this can be done, legally or otherwise, it is difficult to say. The best course for all who read this book, is to be careful, "How to mesmerize, and by whom they are mesmerized."

To alleviate pain and suffering, to cure others of diseases and ailments without drugs or the surgeon's knife, is to engage in work evoking the keenest human sympathy. Here is one of the noblest callings to which humankind can devote its energies— a work of sympathy, love and devotion to our fellow mortals and that science is Mesmerism and Hypnotism; by its influence you can cure diseases and extend powerful influence over the mind of others without their knowledge.

This book is now left to tell its own tale and, with all its faults, it may repay careful perusal.

CHAPTER I.
LIFE OF F. A. MESMER.

Friedrich (or Franz) Anton Mesmer was born at Weil, near the point at which the Rhine leaves the lake of Constance, on May 25, 1733. He studied medicine at Vienna under the eminent masters of that day, Van Swieten and De Haen, took a degree, and commenced practice. Interested in Astrology, he imagined that the stars exerted an influence on beings living on the earth. He identified the supposed force with electricity, and then with magnetism; and it was but a short step to suppose that stroking diseased bodies with magnets might effect a cure. He published his first work (*De Planetarum Influxu*) in 1766.

Ten years later on meeting with Gassner in Switzerland, he observed that the priest effected cures without the use of magnets, by manipulation alone. This led Mesmer to discard the magnets and to suppose that some kind of occult force resided in himself by which he could influence others. He held that this force permeated the universe and more especially effected the nervous systems of men. He removed to Paris in 1778, and in a short time the French capital was thrown into a state of great excitement, by the marvellous effects of mesmerism. Mesmer soon made many converts; controversies arose; he excited the indignation of the medical faculty of Paris, who stigmatised him as a charlatan; still the people crowded to him. He refused an offer of 20,000 francs from the Government for the disclosure of his secret, but it is asserted that he really told all he knew privately to any one for 100 louis. He received private rewards of large sums of money.

Appreciating the effect of mysterious surroundings on the imaginations of his patients, he had his consulting apartments dimly lighted and hung with mirrors; strains of soft music occasionally broke the profound silence; odours were wafted through the room; and the patients sat round a kind of vat in which various chemical ingredients were concocted or simmered over a fire, Holding each other's hands, or joined by cords, the patients sat in expectancy, and then Mesmer, clothed in the dress of a magician glided amongst them, affecting this one by a touch, another by a look, and making "passes" with his hands towards a third. The effects were various, but all were held to be salutary. Nervous ladies became hysterical or fainted; some men became convulsed, or were seized With palpitations of the heart or other bodily disturbances. The Government appointed a commission of physicians and members of the Academy of Sciences to investigate these phenomena; Franklin and Baillie were members of this commission, and drew up an elaborate report admitting many of the facts, but contesting Mesmer's theory that there was an agent called animal magnetism, and attributing the effects to physiological causes. Mesmer himself was undoubtedly a mystic; and, although the excitement of the time led him to indulge in mummery and sensational effects, he was honest in the belief that the phenomena produced were real, and called for further investigation. For a time, however, animal magnetism fell into disrepute; it became a system of downright jugglery, and Mesmer himself was denounced as a shallow empiric and imposter. He Withdrew from Paris, and died at Mearsburg in Switzerland on the 5th March 1815. He left many disciples the most distinguished of whom was the marquis De Puysegur. This noble man revolutionized the art of mesmerism by showing that many of the phenomena might be produced by gentle manipulation causing sleep, and without the mysterious surroundings and violent means resorted to by Mesmer. The gentler method was followed successfully by Deluze, Bertrand, Gearget, Rostan and Foissac in France and by Dr. John Elliotson in England up to about 1830, In 1845 considerable attention was drawn to the announcement by

Baron Von Reichenbach of a so-called new "imponderable" or "influence" developed by certain crystals, magnets, the human body, associated with heat, chemical action, or electricity, and existing throughout the universe, to which he gave the name of Odyl. Persons sensitive of odyl saw luminous phenomena near the poles of magnets, or even around the hands or heads of certain persons in whose bodies the force was supposed to be concentrated.

In Britain an impetus was given to this view of the subject by the translation in 1850 of Reichanbach's Researches on magnetism, in relation to Vital Force, by Dr. Gregory, professor of chemistry in the University of Edinburgh. These researches show many of the phenomena to be of the same nature as those described previously by Mesmer and even long before Mesmer's time by Swedenborg. The idea that some such force exists has been a favourite speculation of scientific men having a mental bias to mysticism, and it makes its appearance not unfrequently.

The next great step in the investigation of these phenomena was made by James Braid, a surgeon in Manchester, who in 1841 began the study of the pretensions of animal magnetism or mesmerism, in his own words, as a "complete sceptic" regarding all the phenomena. This led him to the discovery that he could artificially produced "a peculiar condition of the nervous system induced by a fixed and abstracted attention of the mental and visual eye on one subject, not of an exciting nature." To this condition he gave the name of neuro-hypnotism; for the sake of brevity, neuro was suppressed, and the term Hypnotism came into general use. Braid read a paper at a meeting of the British Association in Manchester on 29th June 1842, entitled Practical Essay on the Curative Agency of Neuro-hypnotism; and his work Neuryphology, or the Rationale of Nervous Sleep considered in relation with Animal Magnetism, illustrated by nervous cases of its successful application in the relief and cure of disease, was published in 1843.

It is necessary to point this out, as certain recent continental writers have obtained many of Braid's results by following his methods and have not adequately recognised the value of the work done by him forty years ago. Braid was undoubtedly the first to investigate the subject in a scientific way, and to attempt to give a Physiological explanation. In this he was much aided by the Physiologist Herbert Mayo and also by Dr. William B. Carpenter,—the latter being the first to recognise the value of Braid's researches as bearing on the theory of the reflex action of ganglia at the base of the brain and of the cerebrum itself, with which Carpenter's own name is associated.

Recently the subject has been reinvestigated by Professor Weinhold of Chemnitz, and more particularly by Dr. Rudolf Heidenhain, professor of physiology, in the university of Breslau, who has published a small but interesting work on Animal Magnetism. In this work Heidenhain attempts to explain most of the phenomena by the physiological doctrine of inhibitory nervous action, as will be shown hereafter.

Phenomena and physiological explanation.—The usual method of inducing the Mesmeric or Hypnotic state is to cause the person operated on to state fixedly at a faceted or glittering piece of glass held at from 8 to 15 inches from the eyes, in such a position, above the forehead as well strain the eyes and eyelids. The operator may stand behind the patient, and he will observe that the pupils are at first contracted from the effort of accommodation of each eye for near vision on the object; in a short time the pupils begin to relax, and then the operator makes a few "passes" over the face without touching it. The eyelids then close; or the operator may gently close them with the tips of the fingers, at the same time very gently stroking the cheeks. Often a vibratory motion of the eyelids may be observed when they are closed, or there may be slight spasm of the eyelids. The eyes may afterwards become widely opened. The patient is now in a sleep-like condition, and the limbs often remain in almost any position in which the operator may place them, as in a cataleptic condition. At the same time the patient may now be caused to make movements in obedience to the commands of the operator, and to act according to ideas suggested to him. Thus, he may eat a raw onion with gusto, apparently under the impression that it is an apple; he may make sad faces on drinking a glass of water when told that what he is taking is castor oil, he may ride on a chair or stool as in a horse race; he may fight With imaginary enemies, or show tokens of affection to imaginary friends; in short, all kinds of actions, even of a ridiculous and a degrading nature, may be done by the patient at the command of the operator. Another class of phenomena consists in the production of stiffness or rigidity of certain muscles or groups of muscles, or even of the whole body. For example, on stroking the forearm it may become rigid in the prone or supine condition; the knee may be strongly bent, with the muscles in a state of spasm; the muscles of the trunk may become so rigid as to allow the body to rest like a dog, head and heals on two chairs, so stiff and rigid as to bear the weight of the operator sitting upon it; or various cataleptic conditions may be induced and as readily removed by a few passes of the hand. Many disorders of sensation have been observed, such as defective colour perception, the hearing of social sounds which have no objective existence, or deafness to certain tones, or perverted sensations, such as tingling, prickling, rubbing, &c, referred to the skin. The patient may remain in this condition for an hour or more, and may then be roused by holding him for a few minutes, and blowing gently into the eyes. Usually, the patient has a vague recollection, like that of a disturbed dream, but sometimes there is an acute remembrance of all that has happened, and even a feeling of pain at having been competed to do ridiculous actions. Certain persons are more readily hypnotized than others, and it has been observed that, once the condition has been successfully induced, it can be more easily induced a second time, a third time more easily than a second and so on until the patient may be so pliant to the will of the operator that a fixed look or a wave of the hand, may throw him at once into the condition. Such are the general facts in artificially induced hypnotism, and they belong to the same class as those referred to animal magnetism, electro-biological effects, odylic influences, &c., according to the whim or theory of the operator. It is not surprising that such phenomena have been the cause of much wonder and the basis of many superstitions. Some have supposed that they were supernatural, others that they indicated the existence of a specific force exerted by the experimenter upon the passive subject. Many operators have no doubt believed they possessed such a force such a belief would not affect the success of their experiments except to make them likely to be successful, as the operator would readily comply with all the conditions; but most of these phenomena can be explained physiologically, and those which cannot be so accounted for will remain hidden until we get further light on the physiology of the nervous system.

The symptoms of the hypnotic state, as shown by Heidenhain, may be grouped under four heads: —

(1) Those referable to conditions of the senroriune or portions of the brain which receives nervous impulses, resulting in movements of a reflex and imitative character;

(2) Insensibility to pain, and various forms of perverted sensation;

(3), Increased irritability of the portion of the nervous system devoted to reflex actions; and

(4) States of the nervous centres controlling the movements of the eye, and accommodation of the eye to objects at various distances, and the movement of respiration, &c.

The state of the sensorium.—By the sensorium is meant that portion of the nervous system which receives impulses from the nerves coming from the organs of sense, such as those from the eye, ear, nose, tongue and skin. Each of these nerves brings its message to a portion of the central nervous system in intimate connection with the rest of the nervous actions of consciousness may be so transient as to leave a fain impress on the memory, so that it can be revived only if no great interval has elapsed since the impression was made on the sense organ If, however, the impression be vivid, then it may be revived long afterwards. This impression may be consciously perceived, and then any apparent effect may end; but it may set up a set of actions, resulting in motion, which are apparently of a reflex character. Thus, suppose a person in the dark; light is suddenly brought before the eye; this affects the retina, and through the changes in it the optic nerve and central organ, there may be consciousness or there may not; if the person be wide awake he will see the light; if he be asleep he will not see it, at all events he will give no indication of seeing it; on awaking, he may have a recollection of a dream in which light has a place, or his memory may be blank; but nevertheless the light will cause the pupil of the eye to contract by reflex action without his consciousness; and perhaps, also without consciousness, the sleeping person may make an effort to avoid the light, as has been noticed in the case of somnambulists. Now, when a patient has been thrown into a weak hypnotic state, there may be a mind recollection on awaking of all that happened during the apparent sleep. This implies, of course, that conscious sensory perceptions took place during the condition. Memory depends on the direction of the attention to sensations. If the effort of attention be strong, the recollection will probably be vivid, and the converse is true. But this does not preclude the supposition that sensory perceptions may come and go, like the shadows of clouds on a landscape without any attempts at fixing them, and consequently with no recollection following their occurrence. The sensory perceptions may have existed for so short a time as to leave no impress behind. This may explain how it is that in the deeper forms of hypnotism there is either no recollection of what occurred or the recollection can only be aroused by hints and leading questions. Attention is necessary, therefore, to form a conscious idea arising out of a sensation.

It is generally admitted by physiologists that the cerebral hemispheres are the seat of the higher mental operations, such as attention, &c., although the interdependence of these hemispheres with the lower sensory ganglia, which receive all sensory impressions in the first instance, and with motor ganglia, which are, in like manner, the starting points of motor impulses, is not understood. The one portion of the nervous system may work without the other. Thus during free cerebral activity we pay little attention to what we see or hear, and consequently we remember nothing. A man in a reverie may have many impressions of sight or of hearing of which he has been really unconscious. On the other hand the cerebral apparatus may be so attuned with the recipient portion that if the latter receives a message the former sympathetically responds. For example, a mother's sound sleep is disturbed by the slightest cry of her child, although loud sounds of other kinds may not awake her.

It would appear then that impressions on the senses and the consciousness of impression are two separate states which may occur in a manner independently; that is to say, there may be purely sensory operations, in which consciousness is not involved, or there may be the conscious repetition of old impressions or what is called memory. Now it is a law of nervous action that processes which at first are always of a conscious kind may by repetition become so habitual as to be performed without consciousness. Thus a child learns to perform a piece of music on the pianoforte by conscious efforts, often of a painful kind; each note has to be recognised and the appropriate muscular movements required for its production on the instrument executed with precision and delicacy; but by and by the music may be performed accurately even while the attention is directed to something else. In like manner, all movements which are the results of sensory impressions may become unconscious movements; the sensory impressions are at first paid attention to; but as they become habitual the mind becomes less and less engaged in the process, until the movements resulting from them are practically unconscious.

A familiar illustration is that of a man in deep reverie, walking, along a street. Immersed in thought, he pays little or no attention to passersby; as his eyes are open, their images, or those of adjacent objects, must affect his visual apparatus, but they arouse no conscious impression and still those impressions evanescent as they are sufficient to excite the appropriate movements of locomotion. These movements are in all respects like voluntary movements but they are not really voluntary showing that by the machinery of the nervous system, movements like voluntary movements may be executed without volition. It is important to observe, however, that these movements are the result of sensory impression. A man in the deepest reverie with his eyes blindfolded, could not execute the requisite movements; and when we see the blind walking in the streets, they afford no contradiction to this view, as their minds are busily engaged in noticing another set of sensory impressions derived from the sense of touch, muscular movement, and hearing, a set of impressions of the greatest importance to them, although of little importance comparatively to ordinary people, who are guided chiefly by visual impressions.

A person in a state of hypnotism may be regarded as in a condition in which the part of the nervous apparatus associated with conscious perception is thrown out of gear, without preventing the kind of movements which would result were it really in action. Impressions are made on the sensory organs; the sensory nerves convey the impressions to a part of the brain; in the deepest condition of hypnotism, these impressions may not arouse any consciousness, but the result may be the kind of movement which would naturally follow supposing the person had been conscious. The movements made by the hypnotic are chiefly those of an imitative kind. It has often been noticed that the mere suggestions of the movement may not be enough to excite it; to secure success, the movement must be made before the eyes of the person. For example, it is a common part of the exhibition of such persons for the operator to clench his fist, the patient at once clenches his; the operator blows his nose; the patient does likewise; but if the operator performs these actions behind the back of his patient the chances are that the patient will not repeat the movements.

The condition seems to be one which the sensory impression leads to no conscious perception and to no voluntary movements, but is quite sufficient to arouse those nervous and muscular mechanisms Which lead to unconscious imitation. The patient is in a sense an automation played upon by the operator through the medium of the patient's sensory organs. It is important to observe that in deep hypnotism the patient has no idea corresponding to the movements he makes in obedience to the example of the operator. For example, suppose he is swallowing a glass of water and the operator tells him it is castor oil, at the same time making the requisite grimaces, the patient will imitate these grimaces without having any idea either of water or of castor oil The grimaces are purely imitative, without any connection with the idea which would naturally excite them. This is the case only with those deeply hypnotized. In some cases, however, the hypnotism is so deep as to resemble coma, and in these there is no trace of any sensory impressions or of movements.

In cases where the hypnotism is slight there may be a curious mixture of effects. Here the patient may be partially conscious of the requests made to him, and of the imitative movements executed before his eyes; to some extent he may resist the commands of the operator, he may feel he is being fooled, and yet he may perform many ridiculous actions; and when he awakes he may have a vivid recollection of the events in which he participated. A hypnotised person, in fact, is in a state similar to that of the somnambulist, who acts the movements of a disturbed dreams. There are many degrees of the sleeping state from the profound condition resembling coma to that of the light sleeper who starts with every sound. In some sleeps there are dreams in which the sleeper is so occupied with the phantoms of thought as to pay no attention to external impressions, unless these be sufficiently powerful to awake him, whilst there are other sleeps in which the boundary between the conscious reception of new impressions and the reproduction of old ones is so thin as to permit of a blending of the two. In this kind of sleep a spoken word, a familiar touch, the suggestion of something in keeping with the thoughts of the dreamer are sufficient to change the current of the dream, and even to excite movements. When the ideas of the dreamer cause movements corresponding to these ideas, then the dreamer becomes a comnambulist. He acts the dream; according to the depth of the semi-conscious state will be his capacity for responding to external impressions. Some somnambulists respond to external suggestions readily, others do not; and in all there is almost invariably no recollection of the state. Artificial hypnotism is a condition of the same kind, though usually not so profound.

The question now arises as to how this artificial state may be induced. In one awake and active, all sensory impressions as a rule are quick, evanescent, and constantly renewed. New successions of images and thoughts pass rapidly before the mind during walking, working, eating or in the leisure hours of social life ; but none last so long as to cause fatigue of any particular part of the body. By and by there is a general feeling of fatigue, and then sleep is needed to restore exhausted nature. But if the attention be fixed on one set of sensory impressions, fatigue is much sooner experienced than if the impressions are various in kind and degree. Thus, one or two hours spent at a picture gallery or at a concert, if the attention be devoted to the impressions on the eye or ear, usually cause fatigue. It would appear that the method of exciting hypnotist by causing the patient to gaze at a bit of glass or a bright button depends in the first place on the feeling of fatigue induced. At first there is a dazzling feeling; then the eyes become moist, images become blurred and indistinct, and seem to swim in the field of vision because unsteady and just about this period the ideas do not pass in the mind in orderly sequence, but irregularly as in the few minutes immediately before passing into sleep. At this stage also the pupils become widely dilated and the eyeballs become more prominent than usual. The innervation of the iris must be understood, so as to appreciate the physiological meaning of these changes. The muscular structure of the iris is supplied by two nerves, the third cranial nerve and the sympathetic nerve. If the third nerve be cut the pupil dilates, if the *distal* end of the nerve be irritated the pupil contracts. On the other hand, if the sympathetic nerve be cut the pupil dilates. These experimental facts show that the radiating fibres of the iris which dilate the pupil are under the control of the sympathetic nerve, whilst the circular fibres which contract the

16

pupil are supplied by the third. Further it can be shown that the corpora quadrigemina two ganglionic masses in the brain, are the reflex centres for the regulation of these movements. The optic nerve from the retina supplies the sensory stimulus which causes the pupil to contract. Thus suppose light to be brought before the eye while the pupil is dilated; the retina is affected a stimulus is sent to the corpora quadrigemina along the fibres of the optic nerve, and from the corpora quadrigemina a nervous influence passes along the fibres of the third nerve to the circular fibres of the iris causing the pupil to contract. It is also very probable that the corpora quadrigemina act as reflex centres for nervous, impulses regulating the calibre of the blood-vessels of the eye the vaso-motor nerves.

If we apply these facts to the case of a hypnotised person we find that

(1) the pupil of a hypnotised person contracts energetically when light falls upon the eye, showing that the reflex mechanism is still intact;

(2) just before the hypnotic state is induced the pupil dilates, indicating feeble nervous impulses passing along the third from the corpora quadrigemina;

(3) at first, the eyeballs seem to sink in, but when hypnotism is complete they project in a manner similar to what has been observed in an animal when the arteries supplying the head have been compressed so as to make the brain anaemic or bloodless ; and

(4) the opthalmoscope has not shown any change in the calibre of the blood vessels of the retina in the hypnotic state.

From a consideration of these facts and inference Heidenhain was at first inclined to believe that hypnotism might be due to a reflex influence on the vessels of the brain, causing them to contract so as to permit the passage of only a small quantity of blood, and make the brain anemic. This view, however, had to be abandoned, as the faces of hypnotised persons are usually red, and not pale, as they would be were the asterioles contracted. Further, Heidenhain performed a crucial experiment by giving to his brother nitrite of amyl, which causes dilatations of the vessels by vaso-motor paralysis, when he still found hypnotism could be readily induced, showing that the state was not caused by deficient blood supply.

Heidenhain has advanced another and more probable hypothesis. During the past twenty years a new mode of nervous action, known as inhibitory action has been discovered by physiologists. A good example is supplied by the innervation of the heart. This organ has nervous ganglia in its substance by which its rhythmic contractions are maintained. Further it is supplied by the vagus or pneumogastric nerve and by the sympathetic section of the vagus is followed by quickening of the heart's action, and stimulation of the lower end causes slowing and if the stimulation be strong enough, stoppage of the heart, not, however in a tetanic state (which would be the case if the fibres of the vagus acted directly on the muscular structure of the heart, as a motor nerve) , but in a state of complete relaxation or diastole.

Opposite results follow section and stimulation of the sympathetic fibres. It has been clearly made out that the terminal fibres of both nerves do not act on muscular fibres but on ganglion cells, those of the vagus "inhibiting" or restraining, whilst those of the sympathetic "accelerate", the action of the cells. Inhibition is now known to play an important part in all nervous actions, and it would seem that any powerful impression in a sensory nerve may inhabit or restrain motion. This is strikingly seen in soma of the lower animals. A ligature applied loosely round the thigh of a frog whilst it lies on the back apparently deprives it of all power of motion. The weak sensory stimulation in this case seems to stop voluntary motion.

Pressure on the internal organs of such animals as the rabbit, although gentle, sometimes causes paralysis of the lower or hinder limbs. Again it has been ascertained that, whilst the spinal cord is the chief reflex centre, the reflex activity can be inhibited by impulses transmitted to it from portions of the cerebral hemispheres which are in a state of high activity. It would appear then, that if we suppose one set. of sensory or recipient cells in the brain to be brought into a state of exalted irritability by the preliminary operations of hypnotism the result might be inhibition of the parts devoted to voluntary movement. In like manner, the activity of sensory nerve cells may become inhibited. Thus stimulation of a certain arm by a mustard plaster has been found to lower the sensibility of the corresponding portion of skin on the opposite arm. The theory then offered is that the cause of the phenomena of hypnotism lies in the inhibition of the activity of the ganglion cells of the cerebral cortex the inhibition being brought about by gentle prolonged stimulation of the sensory nerves of the face or of the auditory or optic nerve.

According to this view, the portion of the brain devoted to voluntary movements is as it were thrown out of gear and the movements that follow, in the hypnotic state are Involuntary, and depend on impressions made on the senses of the patient. To understand how this is possible we must now consider shortly some of the views presently held as to the action of the brain. The researches of Hilzig, Fritsch, Feirier, Hughlings, Jackson and many others indicate that certain movements initiated as a consequence of perception, and of the ideas thereby called forth, are due to nervous actions in the grey matter in certain areas on the surface of the cerebral hemispheres and that there is another class of movements which do not require the agency of the cortex of the brain but depend on the activity of deeper centres. These deeper centres are in the optic thalami, which receive sensory impressions from all parts of the skin; the corpora quadrigemina which receive luminous impressions from the retina; and the corpora striata which are the motor centres whence emanate influences passing to the various groups of muscles. No doubt other sensory centres exist for hearing, taste and smell but these have not been dearly ascertained. In the case of conscious and voluntary movements carried out as the result of external impressions, the excitation would pass first to the thalami optici (tactile) or corpora quadrigemina (visual), thence to cerebral hemispheres, where ideas would be called forth and volitional impulses generated; these would then be transmitted downwards through the corpora striata (motor) to the crura cerebri and spinal cord, and from thence to special groups of muscles, thus causing specific movements. Suppose now that the portions of cerebral hemispheres connected with ideation and volition were thrown out of gear, and that a similar sensory impression was made on the person; again the path of nervous impulses would be to the thalami optici (tactile) or corpora quadrigemina (visual), and from thence directly through corpora striata (motor) to crura cerebri and spinal cord, then passing out to muscles, and causing movements as precise as those in the first instance, and apparently of the same character. The difference between the two operations, however, would be this—in the first there would be movements following perception ideation and volition; in the second the same class of movements would be effected by an automatic mechanism without any of the physical operations above alluded to. This theory has the merit of simplicity and is in accordance with most of the facts. The chief difficulty in the way of accepting it is to understand why, if hypnotism be so induced, it is not induced much oftener. One would suppose that, if gazing at a corn and having a few passes made with the hand were sufficient to bring about physiological changes of such importance, men would be oftener hypnotised in daily life than they are. But it is to be remembered that attention is seldom fixed in one subject so long as in the experiment of producing hypnotism. The first occasion the experiment is made, even with so called susceptible persons, the time occupied may be from 10 to 20 minutes, and during that time the attention is on the strain, and feelings of fatigue are excited in the way above described. Again it is well-known that sudden and strong sensory impression often paralyse voluntary action for a time, even in ordinary life, and what is called "presence of mind" really means the power of self-control which prevents the bodily energies being paralysed by strong sensory impressions. A carriage bearing down on a nervous lady in a crowded street may deprive her of all power of movement or she may automatically run here and there in obedience to the shouts of the bystanders; but one with coolness can thread her way among the vehicles without fear or trouble. A hypnotized person is therefore to be regarded as an automation. "To cause him to move his arm, the image of a moving arm must pass over his retina, or an unconscious sensation of motion must be induced through passive movements of his arm.

2. Insensibility to pain.—It has often been noticed that in the mesmerized or hypnotized person there may be complete insensibility to pain, so that deep pricks with a needle are not felt. During deep hypnotism a pin may be run into the hand without pain, but pain will be felt on awaking, and pulling out the pin in the waking state will cause acute pain. It would appear that certain nerves may convey tactile sensibility whilst others convey only painful impressions, and in certain forms of paralysis the patient may have tactile sensibility without pain, or the reverse. In hysterical women, as has been shown by Charcot and others

disorders of sensibility of this kind are not uncommon, indicating changes in the nervous centres.

3. Increased Reflex Spasm of Muscles.—One of the most striking phenomena of the hypnotic state is the case with which certain voluntary muscles may be rendered stiff. For example, if the operator strokes the skin over the biceps muscle in the upper arm, the limb will be at once powerfully fixed and the biceps can be felt stiff and rigid. To understand the physiological explanation offered of this phenomenon it will be necessary shortly to describe the mechanism of reflex arts. If a sensory nerve be irritated at its periphery, say in the skin, a nervous impulse is transmitted to a central nervous organ, such as the spinal cord, and through the agency of nerve cells in this organ impulses are then transmitted by motor nerves to muscles, causing movements, without any operation of the will. Thus a particle of food getting into the larynx irritates sensory nerves of the vagus and there is a reflex spasm of various muscles of expiration causing a violent cough. That such reflex acts not only can occur without the mill, but in spite of it, is shown by the want of control over a sneeze when the nostril is irritated by snuff. Now these reflex centres in the cord are partially under the control of higher centres in the brain. If the agency of the latter be removed, the activity of the cord-centres is increased, and reflex actions are more easily induced. This we have assumed to be the state of the hypnotic. If a portion of his skin be stroked, first one muscle, say the one immediately under the skin stroked will become stiff, then in obedience to law regulating reflex actions, — namely, that they tend to become diffused, according to the strength and duration of the stimulus,— other muscles become rigid, and so on until the whole trunk becomes cataleptic. This phenomenon is well described by Heidenhain. This condition of the muscles is exactly like that in catalepsy, a peculiar nervous disease; and hypnotism may be regarded as an artificial catalepsy.

4. Other Peculiar Nervous Phenomena of the Hypnotic State.—The changes in the eyes have been already alluded to. The pupils dilate, the eyelids open widely, and the eyeballs protrude. Occasionally the upper eyelids droop, so that the eyelids seem closed. It has often been asserted that clairvoyants see with the eyelids, closed, but they are really partially open. The movements of respiration are often quickened from 16 to 30 or 35 per minute, indicating stimulation of the respirator centres in the medulla oblongata. Sometimes the flow of saliva is increased. Hallucinations of sense may occur, though they are rare. One man in the hypnotic state experienced a strong odour of violets.

There is a class of phenomena referred to the hypnotic state of a very doubtful character, in as much as we have to depend entirely on the statements of the person operated on, and no objective tests can be employed. Such, for example, are various disturbances of sensation, hearing with the pit of the stomach more acutely than when the sound is made is the usual ways towards the ear, and the application of the hand of the operator to the body giving rise to profound sleep or dreams, induced dreaming &c. Again it is asserted by Heidenhain and Gritzner that unilateral hypnosis is possible. Thus stroking the left forehead and, temple caused immobility of the right arm and leg.

Charcot has pointed that in certain kinds of hysteria in women there are remarkable unilateral disturbances or. perversions of sensory impression of colour. Phenomena of the same kind have been observed by Cohn, Heidenhain, and others in hypnotized persons. Thus A. Heidenhain became completely colour blind in the eye of the cataleptic side. All colours appeared grey in different degrees of brightness, from a dirty dark grey to a clear silvery grey. These facts are interesting as showing perverted sensation in the particular individual affected, but they throw no light on the condition of hypnotism.

J. Coates, PHD.

It is evident then that animal magnetism or hypnotism is a peculiar physiological condition excited by perverted action of certain parts of the cerebral nervous organs, and that it is not caused by any occult force emanating from the operator. Whilst all the phenomena cannot be accounted for, owing to the imperfect knowledge we possess of the functions of the brain and cord, enough has been stated to show that just in proportion as our knowledge has increased has it been possible to give a rational explanation of some of the phenomena. It is also deair that the perverted condition of the nervous apparatus of hypnotism is of a serious character, and therefore that these experiments should not be performed by ignorant empirics for the sake of gain or with the view of causing amusement. Nervous persons may be seriously injured by being subjected to suck experiments, more especially if they undergo them repeatedly; and it should be illegal to have public exhibitions of the kind alluded to. The medical professions have always been rightly jealous of the employment of hypnotism in the treatment of disease, both from fear of the effect of such operations on the nervous systems of excitable people, and because such practice is in the border land of quackery and of imposture. Still in the hands of skillful men there is no reason why the proper employment of a method influencing the nervous system so powerfully as hypnotism should not be the means of relieving pam or remedying disease.

ANIMAL MAGNETISM

The terms *Animal Magnetism, Electro-Biology, Mesmerism, Clairvoyance, Odylic, or Odic force* and *Hypnotism*, have been used to designate peculiar nervous conditions in which the body and mind of an individual, were supposed to be influenced by a Mysterious force emanating from another person. With the exception of *Mesmerism*, a name given to the phenomena in honour of one of their earliest investigators, F. A. Mesmer, each

24

of these terms implies a theory. Thus the phenomena of Animal Magnetism were supposed to be due to some kind of magnetic force or influence peculiar to living beings and analogous to the action of a magnet upon steel or certain metals; *Electro-Biology*, a more modern term, introduced in 1850 by two American Lecturers, referred the phenomena to the action of Electrical Currents generated in the living body, and capable of influencing electrically the bodies of others, Clairvoyants implied a power of mental vision or of mental hearing, or of a mental production of other sensations, by which the individual became aware of events happening in another part of the world from where he was, or could tell of the existence of objects which could not affect at the time any of his bodily senses ; odylic force was a term given to a force of a mysterious character by which all the phenomena of animal magnetism might be accounted for; and *Hypnotism*, from "Hypnos" sleep was a name applied to a condition artificially produced in which the person was apparently asleep and yet obedience to the will of the operator as regards both motion and sensation.

HISTORY.—It was natural that the apparent power of influencing the bodies and minds of others should attract much attention and be eagerly sought after for purposes of gain, or from a love of the marvelous, or for the cure of diseases. Hence, we find that, whilst not a few have investigated these phenomena in a scientific spirit, more have done so as Quacks, and Charlatans who have thrown discredit on a department of the physiology of man of the deepest interest. Recently, however, as will be shown in this article, physiologists and physicians have set about investigating the subjects in such a manner as to bring it into the domain of exact science, and to dispel the idea that the phenomena are due either to any occult force or to supernatural agency. It would appear that in all ages, diseases were alleged to be affected by the touch of the hand of certain persons, who were supposed to communicate a healing virtue to the sufferer. It is also known that among the Chaldarans, the Babylonians, the Persians, the Hindus, the Egyptians, the Greeks and the Romans many of the priests effected cures or threw people into deep sleeps in the shades of the temples; during which the sleeper sometimes had prophetic dreams and that they otherwise produced effects like those now referred to animal magnetism. Such influences were held to be supernatural, and no doubt they gave power to the priesthood. In the middle of the 17th Century there appeared in England several persons who said they had the power of curing diseases by stroking with the hand. Notable amongst these was Valentine Greatrakes, of Affane in the Country of Waterford, Ireland, who was born in February 1628, .and who attracted great attention in England by his supposed power of curing the kings evil, or Scrofula. Many of the most distinguished scientific and theological men of the day, such as Robert Bryle and R. Cudworth, witnessed and attested the cures supposed to be effected by Greatrakes, and thousands of sufferers crowded to him from all parts of the kingdom. Phenomena of a marvellous kind, more specially such as imply a mysterious or supernatural power exercised by one person over another, not only attract attention, but take so firm a hold on the imagination that belief in them breaks out now and again with all the intensity of an epidemic. Thus since the time of Greatrakes, at short intervals, men have arisen who have led the public captive at their will. About the middle of the 18th century John Joseph Gassner, a Roman Catholic priest in *Swabia,* took up the notion that the majority of diseases arose from demoniacal possession, and could only be cured, by exorcism. His method was undoubtedly similar to that followed by Mesmer, and others and he had an extraordinary influence over the nervous systems of his patients. Gassner, however, believed his power to be altogether supernatural and connected with religion.

CHAPTER II. HISTORICAL OUTLINE— MESMERISM *PRIOR* TO MESMER.

The principle called Animal Magnetism or Mesmerism being coeval with man's existence, doubtless lay at the foundation of the otherwise inexplicable, mysterious, and miraculous in the life and religions of ancient people. The following will serve to illustrate—"The Charlatans," says Celsus, "performed extraordinary cures by the mere *apposition of the hands*, and cured patients by *blowing*."

Among the Hebrews and Assyrians these means were resorted to in the cure of disease—"Naaman said, I thought he would stand and *strike his hand* [strike up and down in the original] over the place, and recover the leper" (2 Kings v, H). Spiritual powers, gifts of healing, prophecy, and leadership were also conveyed by the *apposition of the hands*: "The Lord said unto Moses, Take Joshua, the son of Nun, a man on whom is the spirit, and *lay thy hands* upon him. Set him before the priest and congregation, and *ask counsel* for him. *And he laid his hands upon him as the Lord commended*" (Numbers xxvii, 18, 23). "And Joshua was full of the spirit of wisdom, because Moses had laid his hands upon him."

Innumerable passages could be quoted from the sacred books of the Hebrews in support of the practice, some of the effects approximating more to the incidents of Modern Spiritualism than to purdy mesmeric phenomena. These, the curious can look up for themselves.

The prophets of Israel, or *seers,* were consulted in private matters as well as the sacred things. In 1 Samuel (Chap. IX) you will find Saul, son of Kish, consulting Samuel the prophet (paying him a fee too in order that he (Saul) might learn from the seer the whereabouts of his father's asses.

Soothsaying, obsession, trance, visions, and inspiration were all accepted facts among these people. The evil and the good depended on the source. When Ahab, King of Israel, wished to know if he should be successful in war and take Ramoth in Gilead, he assembled his prophets to the number of four hundred. This was considered wrong,—as was also the action of Saul, seeking to know his ultimate destiny and that of his kingdom from the spirit of Samuel. Right or wrong, it is never doubted in the sacred record that Samuel did come back and what he predicted did take place. With the Hebrews, Jehovah not only spoke by prophet, revealed His wishes through the seer, but He communicated with man *during dreams* and in the *visions of the night*, to warn "man of the evil he doeth, and to instruct him on the way he should know."

Healing by the laying on of the hands was common among the Jews, and was practised by the Founder of Christianity and His immediate followers with marvellous results. "Many were astonished that such mighty works were wrought by *His hands*" (Mark vi, 2). "*Lay hands* upon the sick, and they shall recover," (Mark xvi. 18). "The Lord granted signs and wonders to be done by *their hands*" (Acts xiv. 3). As illustrative of what I wish to point out in the light of modern science—held in consistently by professing Christians—Naaman, if cured, was cured by *imagination* or *suggestion*, while the cures of Christ and the apostles are placed in the category of effects which had no *occult* basis other than in the "dominant idea" of the "operator" and the "expectancy" of the subject.

MESMERISM AMONG THE GREEKS.

The Greeks derived most of their customs from India and Egypt. Medicine with them was a species of priestcraft the mysteries of which the initiated could not reveal to the profane without sacrilege. The first Greek physicians, for the cure of their patients, used certain magic processes, which can only be compared to the manipulations of the modern mesmerist.

"The affections suffered by the body," says Hippocrates, "the soul sees quite well with shut eyes." "Wise physicians, even among the ancients, were aware how beneficial to *the blood* it is to make *slight friction with hands* over the body. It is believed by many experienced doctors that *the heat* which oozes out of the hand on being applied to the sick, is highly salutary and suaging. The remedy has been found to be applicable to sudden as well as to habitual pains, and various species of debility, being both renovating and strengthening in its effects. It has often appeared, while I have thus been soothing my patients, *as if there were a singular property in my hands to pull and draw away from the affected parts* aches and diverse impurities, by laying my hand upon the place, and by *extending my fingers towards it.* Thus it is known to some of the learned that health may be implanted in the sick by certain gestures, and by *contact* as some diseases may be communicated from one to another."

According to Strabo, there was between Nepa and Fralea a cavern consecrated to Pluto and Juno, in which the priests slept for the sake of the patients who came to consult them.

According to M. Foissac, the familiar spirit, the demon of Socrates, that interior voice which appraised him of that which was to happen, and of that which he should do, was nothing but a state of crisis or of natural somnambulism with which the godlike genius was frequently affected.

In this I do not agree with M. Foissac. We have no record of Socrates having been in a somnambulistic condition, natural or artificial. It were easier to believe that Socrates had a *demon*, that is— a real sentient (but spiritual) being who communicated with him—as he believed—than accept the foregoing, or conclude with M. Lebut, that Socrates laboured under attacks of temporary insanity. Spiritual influences and spiritual faith were not confined to the Israelites.

MESMERISM AMONG THE ROMANS.

Esculapius delivered oracles *in a dream* for the cure of his patients. He *breathed* on the diseased parts, or allayed pain *by the stroking of his hands* and often, as also did his disciples, threw his other patients into long and refreshing sleeps for the recovery of health.

"I will not suffer persons," say Varro, "to deny that the Sibyl has given men good counsel during her life, and that she left after death predictions which are still eagerly consulted on all difficult emergencies.

It is recorded in St. Justin "that the Sibyls spoke many great things with justice and truth, and that when the instinct which animated them ceased to exist, *they lost the recollections* of all they had declared."

According to Celsus, Asclepiades put to sleep, by *means of frictions*, those affected by frenzy. Where their frictions were prolonged, the patient was plunged into a deep lethargic sleep. Heidenhain's "cutaneous irritations" seem to be the legitimate successors of Asclepiades, frictions. There can be no doubt that the effects produced in these and in similar instances were identical in character with the mesmeric phenomena of to-day.

MESMERISM IN FRANCE.

The modern Frenchman, like his ancient forbear, the Gaul, is particularly susceptible to mesmeric influences. Its present day hypnotic wonders are but the continuation, in another phase, of the higher religious manifestations, which took place amid the mystic surroundings of the Druidic temples. Women brought up and instructed by the Druids, we are informed, delivered oracles, foretold the future, and cured diseases. The accounts given by Tacitus Lampridius, and Vopiscus regarding the Druids, bear testimony to the confidence they had in the accuracy of their predictions. Endowed with extraordinary talents, they (the Druidesses) cured diseases deemed incurable, knew the future, and announced it to the people. In the Middle Ages "The Churches'" observes M. Mialle, "succeeded the temples of the ancients, into which the traditions and processes of magnetism were consigned—the same habits of passing whole nights in them, the same dreams, the same visions, and the same cures, The true miracles performed on the tombs of the saints are recognized by characters which is not in the power of man to imitate; but we must exclude from the list of the ancient legends a multitude of very extraordinary cures where religion and faith interfered only *so far as to produce dispositions eminently favourable to the natural action* of magnetism."

A rigid and critical analysis of the records of the middle ages would be here impossible, if not out of place. It would require a volume merely to name the facts, from the exorcisms of Saint Gregory Thaumaturgus to the convulsionaries of Saint Medard. Some intelligent men, one hundred years before Mesmer, like their compeers of to-day, were disposed to deny the reality of the miraculous, or to attribute their existence to magnetism.

J. Coates, PHD.

"Magnetism," says Von Helmont, "is active everywhere, and has nothing new but the name, it is a paradox only to those who ridicule everything, and who attribute to the power of Satan, whatever they are unable to explain."

In -all times, as well as in all countries, extraordinary things have passed for supernatural from the moment they are no longer admitted of explanation; and it is natural to refer and attribute supernatural things to a divine power. That which is esteemed supernatural and divine so becomes the basis of religion. So we find in Pagan antiquity, in the middle ages, and at the present time these phenomena inextricably mixed up with the history of religion.

Miracles (marvellous cures and misunderstood nervous and mental phenomena) were dethroned by the savant in science and philosophy and attributed to magnetism 200 years ago. Even where similar phenomena occur, and are admitted, magnetism— Dia or Zoo—is totally denied by the savants in the present day, at home or abroad, and "the effects attributed to Animal Magnetism in the past are now produced by '"Neuro-Hypnotism," "reflex action of the cerebral nerves," "cutaneous irritations," "expectancy," "suggestion" "credulity," "imagination," "stupidity," and other infinite "isms" appertaining to the nomenclature of modern science. ANIMAL MAGNETISM, it is assured, is a psychological, mathematical point, without form and void, having a location only in the superstitions of the ignorant.

MESMERISM SUBSEQUENT TO MESMER.

DR. ANTHONY MESMER was born on 5th May, 1734, in a small town called Stein, on the bank of the Rhine. This celebrated man studied medicine, and obtained the degree of doctor at Vienna under Professor Van Swieten and Haen, and became acquainted with the virtues of animal magnetism by seeing the
32

wonderful cures performed by a Father Hehl, a Jesuit priest. About 1750 this young doctor commenced to investigate the matter for himself; and, having satisfied himself of the reality of the cures made, he commenced a series of independent experiments. Father Hehl's cures were supposed to be produced by the subtle influence, or fluid of magnetism, which was imparted to patients from steel plates and magnets prepared and used for the purpose. One day Mesmer, having bled a patient, accidently passed his hand over the cicatrix, or lance puncture, and observed that his hand produced the exact results which had hitherto been produced by the magnets.

Mesmer, from the nature of his inaugural thesis. "On the Influence of the Planets of the Human Body," upon obtaining his degree might be expected to see a relationship between the subtle influence exerted by the loadstone or magnet and that of the human hand, and the adoption by him of animal magnetism, as an adequate theory to cover all the phenomena created or experienced by him, seems to have been a natural and easy conclusion.

Mesmer, having learned the art of curing disease from Father Hehl, applied himself to the cure of disease with "extraordinary success." He left Vienna, and travelling throughout Germany and Switzerland he continued to "work wonders" his cures approximating to the miraculous. Kings and Courtiers, as well as the people, vied with each other for an opportunity to attend his *levees* and partake in his *seances*. In 1778 he started for Paris; here his success in curing disease was so remarkable that the *elite* of society struggled for the privilege of waiting upon him and of learning his art. A society was actually formed for the purpose of acquiring his secret and using it for the cure of disease. Somnambulism and clairvoyance had not yet been developed by his process.

J. Coates, PHD.

MESMER'S THEORY OF ANIMAL MAGNETISM.

"There is a reciprocal action and re-action between the planets, the earth, and animated nature.

"The means of operating this action and reaction is a most fine, subtle fluid, which penetrates everything, and is capable of receiving and communicating all kinds of motions and impressions.

"This is brought about by mechanical, but, as yet, unknown laws."

"The reciprocal effects are analogous to the ebb and flow.

"The properties of matter, and of organization, depend upon reciprocal action.

"This fluid exercises an immediate action on the nerves, with which it embodies itself, and produces in the human body phenomena similar to those produced by the loadstone, that is polarity and inclination. Hence the name ANIMAL MAGNETISM.

"This fluid flows with the greatest quickness from body to body, acts at a distance, and is reflected by the mirror like light, and it is strengthened and propagated by sound. There are animated bodies which exercise an action directly opposite to Animal Magnetism. Their presence alone is capable of destroying the effects of Magnetism. This power is also a positive power.

"By means of Animal Magnetism we can effect an immediate cure of the nervous diseases, and a mediate cure of all disorders; indeed, it explains the action of the medicaments, and operates the crisis.

"The physician can discover by magnetism the manner of the most complicated diseases."

Mesmer had many disciples and ardent followers, among whom were some of the ablest men of the day, such as the Marquis of Puysegure, Caullet de Veaumorel, Petetin, Bergasse, Schelling, Von Humboldt, Ritter, Treveranus, Walther, Hufeland, Echenmayor, Nasse, Ness of Essenback, Francis Bader-Kieser, and Jussifeu, the celebrated botanist.

A Commission of Inquiry was appointed by the French Government. The report in the main confirmed the reality of the phenomena. But the whole was conducted in an unsatisfactory manner. The Commissioners could not agree among themselves as to the basis upon which to begin their investigations. They were, however, more or less agreed to this, that Animal Magnetism was the last thing they would give in to. Jusseu, the botanist already mentioned, a member of the Commission, investigated the subject for himself. He pronounced in favour of Animal Magnetism, adducing a great number of facts in its support.

The French Revolution, rather than any mistakes or vagaries of Mesmer, or the unfavourable report of the Commission of Louis XVI, eclipsed the popularity of Mesmerism in France for a time.

In Prussia the light still burned with a steady and brilliant flame. The Prussian Government appointed Professors of Mesmerism at the various Universities throughout the kingdom and established a hospital for the Magnetic treatment of disease at Jena, the director of which was sent to Switzerland to obtain from Mesmer the requisite instructions. The Scientific Society of Berlin offered a prize of 3300 francs for the best explanation of Mesmeric phenomena while the Governments of Russia, Austria and Bavaria passed laws keeping the Mesmeric method of treatment as well as the medical treatment of patients in the hands of the Faculty.

When the Revolution burst forth in France, subverting law, order and all good, Mesmer returned to his native land, where his time was divided between persuing his favourite science and cultivating his estate. Here he was visited by the most eminent men of the day; and before his death he had the pleasure of seeing his works edited by one of the Professors of the University of Strasburg, and his science triumphant in Berlin, Jena, Bonn, Halle, Tubingen, St. Petersbeurg, Copenhagen, and even in Vienna. In spite of laws and law-givers Animal Magnetism performed, the most wonderful cures. Dr. Malfati, one of the most talented of the physicians in Vienna, adopted Mesmer's system, and practised it with great effect.

Following Mesmer, the most active and intelligent of his converts or followers was the Marquis de Puysegure. He pursued the practice of Mesmerism at his estate at Buzancy, both as a study and recreation. One day, calling at the house of his steward, he referred to what he had seen in Paris, where he had attended Mesmer's lectures. Obtaining permission to mesmerize the steward's daughter to his surprise and delight she was in a very short time thrown into a sleep. He also succeeded, by similar passes, in mesmerising the wife of his game-keeper. *He was now confirmed in his faith*, and became one of the most successful mesmerists of his day. He was the first to discover the mesmeric-somnambulistic condition. It happened in this way. He was mesmerizing a young man for the cure of consumption. While making the requisite passes, the patient fell into a peaceful—sleep—the true mesmeric sleep is exceedingly calm and recuperating. While in this sleep Victor talked with an intelligence rare to the waking condition; and while in that state prescribed the remedies necessary to his recovery. Numerous instances of a like character occurring under the Marquis's influence, he at length published a work on the subject and both on his estate and at Paris devoted much time to Mesmerism for the cure of disease, in which he was eminently successful.

De Puysegure's views as to the cause of the phenomena were a slight modification of those of Mesmer. He held views similar to those who believe in organic electricity and odic force. He believed that his subtle electrical agent pervaded all space, all animated beings, and could be controlled and directed by the will. By its skilful direction clairvoyance and somnambulism could be developed in all.

Mesmerism at last found its way across the channel. Mr. Richard Chenevix, F.R.S., published a series of papers on the subject in the *London Medical* and *Physical Journal* for 1829, entitled, "On Mesmerism, improperly called Animal Magnetism." His experiments attracted the attention of the Faculty—Dr. Elliotson, among others. Baron Dupotet arrived in London about 1831, and commenced a series of experiments—the Baron was a firm believer in Animal Magnetism. These experiments were seen by Dr. Elliotson, who now determined to investigate the subject for himself. The result of the experiments of Dr. Elliotson, which was published in the Lancet, produced a great sensation; and *phenomena, which has been regarded as impossible*, were constantly produced. Prevision, introvision, sympathy, thought transference, and all the extraordinary features of clairvoyance were established.

Writing about this period, Samuel Taylor Coleridge, the poet, says:—"My mind is in a state of philosophical doubt concerning animal magnetism. For nine years it has been before me. I have traced it historically, collected a mass of documents on the subject, have never neglected the opportunity to question eye-witnesses, and my conclusion is that the evidence is too strong for a candid mind to be satisfied of its falsehood, or its solubility, on the supposition of imposture, or casual coincidence."

The medical press teemed with incidents, demonstrations, and experiments. Drs. Elliotson, Ashburner, Spillan, Herbert Mayo, and others contributed. The Rev. Chauncey Hare Townsend published his celebrated tracts in 1840. About 1835, Dr. Esdaile's experiments in Calcutta attracted the attention of the Indian Government. Several hundred cases of severe operations, mostly surgical, were performed on patients in the mesmeric sleep. The evidence on 126 cases (was laid before the Government. In ten cases reported on, six were operated upon without any appearance of pain; one indicated movements suggestive of pain, but declared he felt none; and three could not be put asleep. The commission appointed by the Government consisted of nine medical men and a reporter. The report was conclusive, and entirely in favour of Mesmer. As a result, a mesmeric infirmary was established in Calcutta, and all medical students were to take a six month's course there before completing their curriculum. What English physicians were slow to admit at this time— the possibility of carrying out successful surgical operations while patients were in the mesmeric sleep—was quite common to physicians on the continent.

A Mesmeric Infirmary was erected in London, and handsomely supported by public subscriptions. Dr. Elliotson threw his head and soul into the concern, and brought with him all his ability as a medical man (being a short time previously Professor of the London University). Dr. Elliotson had a greater percentage of cures and a smaller percentage of mortality than any infirmary or hospital in London. By such practical results the curative virtues of mesmerism were upheld in this country. In France, the Academy of Medicine, Paris, in 1831, reinvestigated the subject of mesmerism; the result was a triumph for Animal Magnetism, the report being fully in support of that theory.

In France, Germany, Switzerland, India, and now in Great Britain, Animal Magnetism was placed on a scientific basis. In 1841 M. Le Fontaine, a French man, visited England, and commenced giving public lectures on Mesmerism and exhibitions of its phenomena. While in Manchester, he attracted the attention of Dr. Braid, who was at first disposed to treat M. Le Fontaine's experiments as so much imposture., Eventually he admitted the truth of the phenomena with a new theory of his own, which he called *Hypnotism*. Dr. Braid's experiments were remarkable. Although both he and they were ignominiously ignored by the Medical section of the British Association of Science in 1842, it is only right to say that the individual members of the Association gave Dr. Braid great credit for his researches. Heidenhain and Charcot in some respects follows at a distance Dr. Braid. They merely dispute the theory of Animal Magnetism, and attribute the phenomena to monotony, imitation, touch, and imagination — setting up one theory to refute another. Since Dr, Braid published his work, "Neury-hypnology, or the Rational of the Nervous Sleep," 1843, numerous other authors and lecturers have made their appearance, among the most successful of whom were Spencer T. Hall (the Sherwood Forester, author, poet and physician) and Capt. Hudson, of Swan sea. These two gentlemen, more than any other, created great interest in the subject. Henry G. Atkinson and Miss Martineau added to the public interest by their letters and publications. In Scotland, Darling Lewis, Stone, and J. W. Jackson, as experimenters and lecturers, aroused public attention. There are many living now who were delighted and captivated by the experiments of the gentlemen named.

Mesmerism, by its present-day phenomena, will help us largely to understand past mysteries, none the less real because calm and thoughtful scientific investigation furnishes us with a hypothesis—if not sufficiently adequate to cover the whole ground, at least will lead us to see what can be explained on the natural, or within the realm of law, and not beyond it. But of this each reader must judge for him or herself. One thing is certain. Absolute knowledge of what is possible or not within natural law is not possible to the understanding, unless what is infinite can be apprehended the finite. It is only when man in his arrogance or ignorance declares he has discovered the confines of the natural, that he seeks to explain by the supernatural whatever he esteems not possible within the natural. The learned Athenians were "too superstitious." There learned moderns of whom the same might be said. With some all is *matter, no matter what*; with others all is spirit, matter being its temporary projection on a physical plane— "Chaotic ether atoms reduced to cosmos;" while with others there is the conception and perception of the material and the spiritual— of matter and of spirit—as distinct as death and life — the inorganic and the organic. The spiritual may have its basis in mind, mind in organism, organism in protoplasm. If protoplasm is the physical basis of life and mind in animated nature, what is the vitalizing essential—spirit or what—which is the basis of protoplasm? Shall I say I don't know what matter, or mind, or life, or spirit is? I know not, save by their manifestations. Magnetism—electricity—can neither be defined nor known, only as interpreted by law of manifestation. If we find a *force* in man or in animals analogous in its manifestation, to magnetism in a stone — *i.e.* attractive and repellent forces —polarity—we are justified in calling that force Animal Magnetism for want of a better name. It is in this sense the word is used by mesmerists. The existence of such an influence has been denied, because similar or apparently similar phenomena have been induced by persons who did not believe in Animal Magnetism. That, perhaps, does not amount to much, seeing that these objectors *believed they had and have power to induce the phenomena* by adopting other means. They thus exercise their WILL-POWER and exert their INFLUENCE by their POSITIVE assumption of another hypothesis all the same. I believe in Animal Magnetism. From long practice I have seen much to induce me to realize and demonstrate that man can exercise such a force— a force which, in its nature and character, is no more occult than nerve force, magnetism, light, heat, or electricity. All mesmeric phenomena, it is true, can not be traced to Animal Magnetism. If successfully traced to secondary causes—hypnotism, suggestion, imitation, and what not—it is a matter of really little importance, so long as the whole phenomena can be lifted out of the misty superstitions and vulgar exaggerations of the past and present, out of the darkness of fraud and self-deception, into the light of truth and fact, by investigation and demonstration. In the next chapter I shall deal with "Modes of Procedure."

CHAPTER III.
MODES OF PROCEDURE.

The phenomena presented by persons under the influence of Animal Magnetism or Mesmerism are various, as well as the methods by which the effects are produced. The former are classed under six degrees, as follows. The latter will be presented under Modes of Procedure.

1st Degree.—THE WALKING STAGE.—In which the subject may, or may not, have been affected, although operated upon. It presents no phenomena, the intellect and senses retaining, apparently, their usual powers and susceptibility.

2nd Degree.—THE TRANSITION STAGE.—In which the subject is under Imperfect control, most of the mental faculties retaining their activity. Of the senses, vision is Impaired, and the eye withdrawn from the control of the subject. That may also be termed the sub-hypnotic stage.

3rd Degree.—THE SLEEPING STAGE.—In which the mesmeric sleep, or coma, is complete. The senses refuse to perform their respective functions. The subject is, therefore, unconscious to pain. In this stage he can be catalepsed, and his mind automatically influenced, by whatever position his body may be placed by the operator.

4th Degree.—THE SOMNAMBULISTIC OR SLEEP-WALKING STAGE.—Under which the subject "wakes up", within himself. The faculties become responsive to mesmeric influence, direction, and suggestion, the sensitive becoming largely an irresponsible agent—thinking, seeing and hearing only as permitted or as directed by the mesmerist. It is in this stage that the phenomesmeric and mostly all other experiments are conducted, whether deemed mesmeric or hypnotic. The lower form of the degree is designated by the mesmeric-psychological state.

5th Degree.—THE LUCID SOMNAMBULISTIC STAGE.—In which, in addition to the phenomena indicated in the 4th Degree, that of lucid vision, or *clairvoyance* (including thought-transference, introvision, and prevision), is manifested. In this state the patient is able to obtain a clear knowledge of his own internal, mental, and bodily state, is able to calculate the nature of his, or her disease, prescribe suitable remedies, and foreshadow the termination of attack. The patient placed *en rapport* or in sympathy with a third person, is enabled in their case to exercise the same faculty of internal inspection, diagnosis and ability to prescribe and foreshadow the results of treatment.

6th Degree.—THE INDEPENDENT OR SPIRITUAL STAGE.—In this the patient's vision is not limited by space or sympathy. He passes wholly, as in the last stage partially, beyond the control of the operator.

The phenomena occurring under the first four degrees are exceedingly common to all mesmerists. These of the fifth degree, although not so common, are well authenticated under old mesmeric processes. They have not been produced under the now-popular hypnotic method. The sixth degree, although rare, is wen substantiated by the best authorities on the subject. The fifth and sixth degrees seem to indicate that man has a soul, or spiritual existence, or that he is a *spirit even now*, although clothed in a body. This idea is rejected by many of our leading men of science and by all materialists. *Spirit* is about "the last thing they can give in to." Their thoughts and conceptions of things are, of necessity, largely moulded by their favourite studies and pursuits in the physical and material.

The stages described are not progressive and developed in sensitives in the order indicated, but rather, states produced according to the temperamental condition or peculiarities of organism in persons operated upon, the majority of whom never pass the fourth stage. All phases may be developed in one subject; some may pass rapidly into the fifth or sixth stage without apparently having passed through the others. Some subjects seem to have a natural fitness for one class of phenomena and not another. Those adapted for the higher phases of thought transference, or sympathetic thought-reading, would be degraded or injured (that is, their powers obscured), were they reduced to the buffooneries of the public platform; while those most suited for public entertainments, seldom or never are fitted for the exhibition of the higher stages of the fourth degree, and certainly never for the fifth and sixth. This explains why the phenomena of the higher degrees have been so fugitive or unreliable. Mesmerists, straining for effect, or carried away by some previous successes, have endeavoured to reproduce them, and, in doing so, have injured their sensitives, not knowing that these phenomena depend more upon certain nervous and psychic conditions in the sensitive, than in the mesmeric powers of direction possessed by the operator.

I mention the foregoing as a warning and a precaution. Mesmerists should bring the sobriety of calmness—a scientific watchfulness—into all their operations. They should always remember that, while their *influence*, according to the adaptability, may predispose to the *development* of the higher phases of the phenomena in their subjects, it is only a development—the faculties must be innate in the latter, by which the phenomena are expressed.

MODES OF PROCEDURE.

Having thus briefly pointed out the various recognised stages of phenomena, I shall now glance at the Modes of Procedure successfully adopted by various operators. The first of these are the mesmerists who accept the theory of *nervous fluid*; susceptible of being influenced and producing an influence, as the primary operating agent in these phenomena. Next are the Hypnotists, an important class, of whom Dr. Braid, of Manchester, was the founder. There is much to be said in favour of his views. A full explanation of them would be too tedious and technical for a work of this wind. To his credit, it must be said, he was the first who did justice to the individuality or personal powers of the sensitive. He reproduced many of the effects induced by mesmerists without, what he denied, mesmeric influence or the influence of a second person, and accounted for the phenomena by supposing that there is a derangement of the cerebro-spinal centres and of circulating and respirating and muscular systems, induced by a fixed state, absolute repose of body fixed attention and suppressed respiration, concurrent with fixity of attention." Also he expressed his opinion "that the whole depended on the physical and psychical condition of the patient, arising from the causes referred to, and not at all on the volition or passes of the operator throwing out a magnetic fluid or exciting into activity some mystical universal fluid or medium." Had Mr. Braid been living now he would have been surprised to see how his ideas have been developed in certain quarters, and that with very chary acknowledgment to himself.

Following Braid, Dr. Rudolph Heidenhain, Professor of Physiology at the University of Breslau, stands next highest in order of Hypnotists. After Heidenhain, and contemporary with him as a specialist, was the late Dr. Carpenter. He placed Mesmerism and Spiritualism in the same category, and accounts for the whole of the phenomena said to occur in connection with either to "unconscious mental cerebration," "dominant ideas," and "expectancy."

Closely following Heidenhain and Dr. Carpenter came include in their practice the suggestions and methods of Braid, Heidenhain and Carpenter.

The methods adopted by mesmerists in a large degree vary. Each operator will have his own special mode. Some of these may be of interest, and help those who may possibly undertake to experiment on their own account.

However, let none lightly enter upon the task, unless they are adapted for the work. Many persons have very foolishly done so—commenced to try experiments with no other knowledge than that of having seen some other person's experiment. Some years ago I gave a successful series of demonstrations at the Queen's Rooms, Bold Street, Liverpool. A gentleman residing in Bootle was present with his family one evening. On returning home he thought, for the "fun of the thing," he would "try his hand." He had no doubt that he could do just as well as myself, as he afterward told me. He succeeded in putting his footman asleep, and of getting him to do several things, which he (the gentleman), his family, and servants enjoyed amazingly. He was in raptures with his more than expected success, the subject being exceedingly passive and docile in his hands. He however, forgot how to de-mesmerise, or wake the subject up. Becoming perplexed and excited, the poor footman followed suit. One person suggested one thing, another, another thing. This gentleman tried to carry out the various suggestions, but the poor victim was fast retrograding from bad to worse. Smelling salts were applied to his nose and water thrown over him; these efforts only unduly excited him. He groaned and cried, and acted in a very strange manner. A messenger was sent into town; at considerable trouble I was found, and at four o'clock in the morning arrived at his house. I saw how things stood, and proceeded to de-mesmerise his footman by the following process: —I got every person in the house who had touched the young man to take hands and join in a circle, the gentleman who had mesmerised the youth taking his (the footman's left hand, while I completed the circle by taking his right hand. I counselled passivity and calmness on all, and explained to them the risk of indiscriminating experiments, and the dangers which might arise therefrom, and pointed out that this was a bad case of "Cross-Mesmerism." By forming the circle, I sought to tone down the tumult, calm the patient, and subject all to my own influence. At the end of fifteen minutes I broke up the circle, placed myself in dominant contact with the patient, and de-mesmerised him. The lesson was not readily forgotten by either the gentleman or his servants. The former had a course of instruction, and became afterwards a very successful mesmerist.

DELAUZES MODE OF PROCEDURE.

Using his own words, "Once you will be agreed and determined to treat the matter seriously, remove from the patient all those persons who might occasion you any restraint, do not keep with you any but the necessary witnesses (only one if possible), and require of them not to interfere by any means in the *processes* which you employ and in the *effects* which are the consequences of them, but to combine with you doing good service to the patient.

"Manage so as to have neither too much heat nor cold, so that nothing may constrain the freedom of your movements, and take every precaution not to be interrupted during the sitting.

"Then take your patient, sit in the most convenient manner possible opposite to him, or her, on a seat somewhat higher, so that his knees may be between yours, and that your feet may be between his. First, require him to resign himself, *to think of nothing*, not to distract his mind in order to examine the effects he will experience to banish every fear to indulge in hope, and not to be uneasy or discouraged if the action of *magnetism* produce in him momentary pain. After matters are well adjusted, take his thumbs between your two fingers, so that the interior of your thumb may touch the interior of his, and fix your eyes on him. You will remain from two to five minutes in this position, until you feel that an *equal heat* is established between his thumbs, and yours. This being done, you will draw back your hands, separating them to the right and left, and turning them so that the inner surface may be on the outside, and you will raise them a little higher than the head, then you will place them on the two shoulders, you will leave them there for about a minute, and you will bring them down the arms as far as the ends of the fingers, slightly touching them You will recommence the pass five or six times turning away your hands and separating them a little from the body, so as to re-ascend. You will then place your hands above the head; you will keep them there for a moment, and you will bring them down, passing in front of the face, at the distance of one or two inches, as far as the pit of the stomach; there you will stop for about two minutes, placing your thumbs on the pit of the stomach and the other fingers below the ribs. Then you »will descend slowly along the body as far as the knees, or better and if you can without incommoding yourself, to the extremity of the feet. You will repeat the same process during the greater part of the sitting; you will also approach the patient sometimes, so as to place your hands behind his shoulders, and let them descend slowly along the spine to the back, and from thence on to the haunches and along the thighs so far as the knees, or even to the feet. After the first pass you may dispense with placing the hands on the head, and make the subsequent passes on the arm. If no results are produced in half-an-hour, the sitting terminates, and the foregoing process is repeated again. The desired results will take place at the end of the second or of some subsequent sitting.

Slow work, one would think; yet this is a fair specimen of the older methods of operating, and one from which the best results accrued. One of the great secrets of mesmeric success is indomitable perseverance, patience, and capacity for slow, plodding work.

MR. COLQUHOUN'S MODE OF PROCEDURE.

This gentleman's method and explanations are exceedingly interesting. He says, "The magnetic treatment is usually administered with the hand, and is thence called manipulation. The usual method is to stroke repeatedly with the palms of the hands and fingers in one direction, downwards from the head to the feet; and in returning to throw the hands round in a semi-circle, running the palms outside in order not to disturb the effects of the direct stroke. To magnetize in the contrary direction, that is from the feet upward towards the head, not only counteracts the effects of the former method, but frequently operates of itself prejudicially, especially in the case of irritable subjects. If we attempt to operate with the back of the hands, no effect whatever will probably be produced upon the patient. "If, in the course of this process, the hands or fingers of the operator are made actually to touch the body of the patient, it is called manipulation with contacts if on the contrary, the operation is conducted at some distance, it is called manipulation in distance. The manipulation with contact is of two kinds; it is accompanied either with considerable pressure or with light touching—manipulation with strong or with light contact. The manipulation with strong universally prevalent mode of operating". In my experience the best results have been produced by passes at distance and by light contact. Any other treatment of fine subjects and sensitive patients would unduly excite nervous irritation and cerebral activity. This must be avoided if the object of the passes is to produce sleep, alleviate pain, or cure disease.

CAPT. JAMES' MODE OF PROCEDURE.

It affords me great pleasure to reproduce the remarks of this gentleman. Personally, I consider that Captain James was the most successful mesmerist since the days of Dr. Elliotson, whose friend and pupil he was. This gallant British officer served his country in the 90th Light Infantry and had many opportunities of witnessing and testing mesmeric phenomena at home and abroad. Such personal acquaintance as I fortunately had with this gentleman convinced me, he was a man of the most sterling character, intellectual and moral—one imbued not only with a strong sense of honour, but a deep and compassionate sympathy for suffering, kindly and unpretentious in all his ways. He never was a *public mesmerist*, and all the good he did—in a large, wide and well-known circle—was a *free gift*—a worthy pupil of a noble tutor, truly.

He writes—"It is recommended that the mesmerist should direct his patient either to place himself in an easy-chair, or lie down on a couch, so that he may be perfectly at ease. The mesmerist then, either standing or seated opposite his patient, should place his hand, with extended fingers, over the head, and make passes slowly down to the extremities, as near as possible to the face and body without touching the patient, taking care at the end of each pass to close his hand until he returns to the head, when he should extend his fingers and proceed as before. It is also useful, after making several of these passes, to point the fingers close to the patient's eyes, which procedure in many cases, has more effect than the passes. This simple process should be continued for about twenty minutes at the first seance, and may be expected to produce more or less effect according to the susceptibility of the patient. Should the operator perceive any signs of approaching sleep, he should persevere with the passes until the eyes dose, and should he then observe a quivering of the eyelids, he may be pretty certain that his efforts will be successful.

"Sometimes slow breathing, or placing the hand on the forehead, will deepen the sleep; but the beginner should, as a rule, avoid concentrating the mesmeric force on the head or region of the heart, and confine himself as much as possible to the passes, *aux grands courants* as the French writers term them, the long slow passes from the head to the feet. Should the above described signs of mesmeric coma not declare themselves at the end of twenty or thirty minutes, the mesmerist should ask the patient whether he felt any peculiar sensation during the process, and if so, whether they were more apparent during the passes or when the fingers were pointed at the eyes. By these inquiries he will soon learn the best method of mesmerising applicable to each particular case, and he should not be disheartened if he does not succeed in producing marked effects at the first or even after successive seances. Pain may be removed and diseases cured or greatly alleviated without the production of sleep, and many patients succumb at length who have for many weeks been apparently unaffected and proof against all the resources of the mesmerisers.

"Supposing sleep to be at length induced, the next and very important question is how to awaken the patient. With most sensitives this is a very easy process, for merely blowing or fanning over the head and face with a few transverse passes will at once dispel sleep. Should, however, the patient experience a difficulty in opening his eyes, then with the tips of his thumbs the operator should rub firmly and briskly over the eyebrows from the root of the nose outwards towards the temples, and finish by blowing or fanning, taking special care before leaving the patient in that condition judging from the expression of his normal state. As a rule, the patient should not be left until the operator is perfectly satisfied that he is wide-awake.

"There are certain cases, however, where the sensitives should be allowed to sleep for two or three hours, or even more, and particularly when lengthened sleep has been prescribed by the patients themselves. Cure must be taken to ascertain that they can be left alone with impunity. The majority may be; but there are cases where the operator should not be absent during the sleep. With a little observation the mesmeriser should be able to distinguish between such cases, and learn to adapt his treatment according to the peculiar temperament or constitution of each patient.

"Should there be a difficulty in arousing the patient the mesmeriser may frequently bargain with him as to how long the sleep is to last; and should he promise to awake in the course of one or two hours, he will generally fulfil his promise by waking almost at the very minute named. The mesmeriser may also insist that his patient should awake at a certain time, and will in most cases be obeyed.

"This power of acting or impressing the patient's mind may be carried into and continued in the normal or waking state, and might be used with good effect in treatment of dipsomania and other morbid habits so that the patient would in many cases, in consequence of the impressions made during his sleep, be led to entertain an actual disgust at the mere smell of alcoholic liquor.

"The patient during his sleep can frequently give valuable directions to his mesmeriser both as to the best methods of mesmerising him and the most effective means of terminating the sleep. In some rare cases the sleep is so prolonged, in spite of all the operator's efforts to dispel it, that he is alarmed, and the patient becomes affected in his fears. ABOVE ALL THINGS, THE MESMERISER SHOULD PRESERVE HIS PRESENCE OF MIND, and he may be assured that the longest sleep will end spontaneously.

"It may as well be observed in this place that the *patient should not be touched by anyone but his mesmeriser* unless he wish it or at least gives his consent. He can perhaps, bear the touch of certain individuals, and may express a repugnance to be touched by others, and this quite irrespective of attachment or repulsion with regard to those individuals in his normal state. With most sensitives it is quite immaterial who or how many people touch them, but there are occasionally cases when, by so touching them, a very distressing state, called "Cross Mesmerism," is produced, and the more particularly in the case of patients who are naturally highly nervous and, perhaps hysterical. It is in these cases of Cross-Mesmerism that we most often find a difficulty in determining the sleep."

The foregoing is a pretty full extract: I give it because it presents, in the simplest form, the procedure of the best class of mesmerists. The entire absence of technicalities and pedantic language has also much to recommend it to my readers. In it we find that perseverance, diligence, and presence of mind are the essential requisites for a mesmerist; that certain methods of operation are adopted as expressive of the will and determination of the mesmerist to produce certain results; that the phenomena not only vary in different patients, but at different periods in the same patient. The method of awaking, the curative and phenomena of suggestion, or the power of impressions made during sleep, are also faithfully and simply pointed out.

J. Coates, PHD.

HYPNOTISM.

There are several degrees in sleep, and various stages, or *states*, in Mesmerism. So there are different hypnotic states. These are said to be three in number, and, from their characteristics, they approximate in a marked degree to the second, third and fourth stages of mesmerism. By Braid, Heidenhain, Charcot, and Richer these hypnotic states are classified as the CATALEPTIC, the LETHARGIC and the SOMNAMBULISTIC.

In the first, or Cataleptic stage, the subject possesses no volition, does not respond to mental or verbal suggestions,— nervous muscular excitability appears to be absent—and in whatever position the various parts of the body are placed, they will remain in that position.

In the second, or Lethargic stage, the subject is a helpless lump of insanity; the muscles are unflexed, flaccid, and flabby, the eyes are closed, and the body is in all respects like that conditioned by a dead faint, or, in a lesser degree, by the *coma* of drunkenness. Surgical operations can be performed in either stage, without real or apparent pain to the subject.

The third, or Somnambulistic stage, approximates to the fourth degree of Mesmerism. The subject acts as if in a dream,— but he acts the dream— such as may be suggested by the operator. The phenomena elicited in this stage are complex, so much depending on the temperament and phrenological aptitudes of the subject. With good subjects, memory, reflection, and imagination can be intensified and exalted, the past recalled to the present, and action done therein confessed, should such be determined upon by the operator. As in Mesmerism these states vary—may be developed one after the other on the same subject. The majority of hypnotic subjects pass from the cataleptic to the somnambulistic without any apparent intervening condition.

DR. BRAID'S MODE OF PROCEDURE.

I give his plan in his own words: —"Take any bright object (I generally use my lancet case) between the thumb and fore and middle fingers of the left hand; hold it from about eight to fifteen inches from the eyes, at such a position above the forehead as may be necessary to, produce the greatest possible strain upon the eyes and the eyelids, and enable the patient to maintain a steady, fixed stare at the object. The patient must be made to understand that he must keep the eyes steadily fixed on the object. It will be observed that, owing to the consensual adjustment of the eyes, the pupils will be at first contracted, they will shortly begin to dilate, and after they have done so to a considerable extent, and have assumed a very wary position, if the fore and middle fingers of the right hand, extended and a little separated, are carried from the object toward the eyes, most likely the eyelids will close involuntarily, with a vibratory motion. If this is not the case, or the patient allows the *eyeballs too move*, desire him to begin again, giving him to understand that he is to allow the eyelids to close when the fingers are again carried to the eyes, but that the eyeballs *must* be kept fixed on the same position, and the mind riveted to the one idea of the object held above the eyes."

Here we find although Dr. Braid avows that the influence of a second person is not necessary, he exercises his own will in a marked manner. He directs the attention of the patient, gives him to understand he must do something—i.e., in this instance he must steadily gaze on a bright object, so as to "weary the optic nerves and exhaust the muscles of the eyes. Here the will of the operator is exercised in a large measure. His methods induce inhibition of the nerve centres which govern the optic nerve. The control obtained is inferior to the ordinary mesmeric method—it is first physical, and then mental. The subject concludes, unconsciously though it be, and having lost the sense of sight and the control of his own vision, that the operator can do whatever he pleases, and the subject passively, intuitively falls in with the impressions and directions of the operator accordingly. But the results achieved by the best hypnotic processes fall far short of those attained by the older and calmer operations of Mesmerism.

Dr. Braid, being a man who had the courage of his convictions, and therefore just such a person who was most likely to be a successful operator, commenced to investigate the subject with the intention to expose what he esteemed a swindle. The ultimate results of his experiments proved the reality of mesmeric phenomena. He also was obliged to admit that the *hypnotic state* was a new discovery, not identical with the mesmeric sleep or *coma*, but in some measure allied thereto. He found abundant evidence from his own experiments of the reality of an induced state—nervous, mesmeric, or hypnotic sleep—which could be produced artificially; that in that state the senses, with the exception of sight, were wonderfully exalted—for instance, hearing and smell became intensified. "Thus a patient who could not hear the ticking of a watch beyond three feet when awake, could do so when hypnotised at a distance of thirty-five feet, and walk to it in a direct line without difficulty or hesitation. Smell in like manner is so wonderfully exalted that a patient has been able to trace a rose through the air, when held forty-six feet from her."

The reality of the phenomena grew upon this ardent and painstaking investigator and while adhering to his theoretical conceptions, he found in Hypnotism a new and powerful curative agent—rheumatism of ten years standing, deafness, neuralgia, lumbago, spinal irritation, paralysis of sense and motion, St. Vitus' dance, tonic spasm, diseases of the skin, and many other apparently intractable diseases, became obedient to his mystic power and departed. "I am quite certain," he said, "that Hypnotism is capable of throwing a patient in that state in which he shall be entirely unconscious of the pain of a surgical operation, or of greatly moderating it, according to the time allowed and the mode of management resorted to."

Dr. Braid also found that illusions, by impression or suggestion, created in the mind of a subject in the *hypnotic state were always faithfully acted upon in their waking condition.*

PROF. HEIDENHAIN'S MODES OF PROCEDURE

Heidenhain's Modes of Procedure are apparently very simple—1st, such as monotonous stroking of the temples or nose; and, by monotonous sounds such as the ticking of a watch. Experiment as follows: —Professor Heidenhain placed three chairs with their backs against a table, upon which he had previously placed his watch. Three persons sat down' upon the chairs, with their attention directed to the monotonous ticking of the watch, and all three fell asleep. Here again the sleep and any attending phenomena is brought about by acting upon the physical first, the mental following. Dr. Braid wearies the eyes, and exhausts the inferior and lateral muscles. Heidenhain, by the well-known connection of the skin to the nervous system, produces weariness in the censorium—through the inhibition of the sense of feeling—by stroking the skin; of hearing, by the monotonous ticking of the watch. The persons operated upon are necessarily pretty sensitive to his will, expressed by determined suggestion. A sudden fright has been known to produce the hypnotic condition. I have seen a cat catalepsed on a yard-wall by a broom being thrown at it; a thief catalepsed at the sudden fear of detection. Hypnotism is not Mesmerism. In Mesmerism the 5th and 6th degrees previously referred to are frequently induced—in Hypnotism never. In the mesmeric state the senses, as a rule, are temporarily suspended—the subject feels, tastes, or smells in sympathy with or through his mesmeriser; in the hypnotic state the senses are exalted, their power intensified as already described. In the former the mental faculties have a refined, definite, and coherent action; in the latter, as in dreaming, any illusion created by the operator appears to be a reality. In the mesmeric, the sleep is calm, refreshing, and curative, the pulse slow and rhythmic: in the hypnotic state the respiration is frequently irregular, accompanied by slight convulsive movements, nausea and vomiting, and general prostration of the nervous system. Hypnotism is, of course, modified by the temperament, character, and health of the subject; so is Mesmerism, for that matter, but the foregoing out of many observed instances serve to point out the essential difference between the two states. The Hypnotism of Charcot, Mm. Bourru, Butot, Voisin, and others—Heidenhain, for that matter,—are but modifications of the discovery of Dr. Braid. "I do not pretend to say that it (Mesmerism) can never do harm, but I can say that in all cases which I have seen treated myself, of which a great number occurred in nervous individuals affected with various diseases—*even with diseases of heart*, which would appear most liable to suffer from all extraordinary excitation—the effect of magnetic process in general and of sleep in particular has always been calming, and *in no instance* has it been disagreeable to the patient; it acted, moreover, in a beneficial manner upon their health." — Gregory, late Professor of Materia Medica, University of Edinburgh.

I cannot say this about Hypnotism. That it has Its useful and beneficient side must be admitted, yet no power can be more degraded. I never knew Mesmerism, properly applied, do harm. Hypnotism is a coarser form of Mesmerism and is induced by various means, as already indicated.

The mesmeric and the hypnotic states are often confounded with one another, but they are distinct if allied. In the first the subject has an inward illuminated condition—a strong moral and spiritual individuality—a penetration and clear-headedness marked and distinct; in the latter subject is a creature of circumstances, and the circumstances may be good, bad, or indifferent.

CHAPTER IV. MODES OF PROCEDURE.—
(*Continued*)

It is not to be doubted that the various hypnotic methods are capable of producing extraordinary results, whether these methods are those of the inhibition, of nerve centres, by monotonous strokings, sounds, movements, or purdy by *suggestion*, with its varying action and psychological influence, according to the presence, power, and peculiarities of the operator or the temperament and character of the patient or subject. Remarkable as these results may be, and admitted that the methods used to bring them about do in some measure enter occasionally in all mesmeric practice, still the phenomena is never of that beautiful character as those evolved by the slower, more patient and carefully administered methods known as mesmeric.

MAGNETIZING WATER.

There is a subtle life-force in mankind and in animals to which the term Zoo—Organic or Animal Magnetism, or Odic force—has been used to distinguish. This *force or influence*, by whatever name, is the main agent in mesmeric phenomena. I have carefully magnetized a tumbler of water, being one of six tumblers of water. The tumblers were placed on a tray by a committee appointed for the purpose. The patient has, by sight and taste detected the magnetised or mesmeric water from the rest by the sensations experienced by him.

Odylic—of Riechencach.

I have mesmerised flannel, and even paper, for patients at a distance, with satisfactory results, which neither faith, suggestion, nor Psychology can explain. I give one instance out of many. Mr.

J. M., merchant, of Stornoway, paid me a special visit in Liverpool in 1877, and placed before me the case of his father—an old gentleman, troubled with insomnia, or sleeplessness, brought on with commercial troubles and in a large measure, by old age. Everything that kindness, good nursing, and medical skill could do for him had been done, without success. As a *dernier [last] resort*, I was consulted.

I magnetised a large band of flannel, with the intention of producing sleep. It was taken home by J. M., and *sewn into his father's under-garment, unknown to the father*, and put upon him when his night clothes were changed, with the result that in a quarter of an hour after it was put on, he fell into a refreshing slumber of nine hours.

In this instance the person benefited was the under another's *influence*, conveyed by the means of a piece of flannel. In this case disease had rendered the person benefited peculiarly susceptible to the *influence*. Another person not so situated might not have experienced any influence at all.

The experiments of Braid, Heidenhain, Charcot; Carpenter, and others certainly go far to prove their own respective theories, and do in a measure dethrone Animal Magnetism. But these gentlemen forgot that their experiments are not mathematical researched, in which the tendency of error is reduced to a minimum. Their experiments, on the contrary, have been with variable quantities—fugitive and psychological—and which must in the nature of things be influenced by predominate ideas of the experimenters. W. H. Myers, M.A., of London, one of the most learned of living investigators of occult phenomena, says: "I still hold to the view of Cuvier, that there is in some special cases a specific action of one organism on another of a kind as yet unknown. This theory is generally connoted by the term "Mesmerism."

Some of the most ardent of recent hypnotists are beginning to admit the possibility of some special agent or influence on these phenomena. Dr. Siebault, of Nancy—one, perhaps, of the ablest of living hypnotists, and one who at one time was disposed to deny the possibility of such an *influence*—has, at the end of 25 years, during which time he has hypnotised or magnetised thousands of persons in health and disease, arrived at the conclusion that such specific influence does exist, which he terms "Zoo-Magnetism."

I should advise all experimenters to act as is such influence existed. That in every move and pass, look or gaze, act as if they were throwing out something, or imparting that something with a definite end in view, all looks and passes being but vehicles to conduct the specific influence. By use of the term mesmeric, I include the possibility of such an influence, the means of applying and conducting it, and all such means or aids as will assist in intensifying it, or will aid in bringing about the desired result in conjunction with it, such as suitable conditions, and even the aid of imitation, suggestion, and imagination. If these latter can be used to good purpose, why not use them?—if not, why not?

In 1880 I was engaged in Glasgow to attend a case in Uddingston. The gentleman had been professionally engaged for many years abroad. Through ill health he had to return home to Scotland. Shortly after his arrival, he took seriously ill, seemed to lose all hold upon life and interest therein. His case was complicated by sleeplessness. Here, again, medical skill had applied every known means to give relief. Bromides and chlorals, draughts and subcutaneous injections, seemed to intensify his sufferings and wakefulness, instead of giving relief. I was engaged by the direction of the family physician and the consulting professor. I found for six weeks he had little or no sleep, and the patient was very weak, nervous, and irritable. A friend of the family had tried monotonous sounds—namely reading slowly page after page of an uninteresting book, in a most lullaby fashion; all no use, I commenced operations at the bedside at ten, and the patient was soundly asleep at eleven. In a fortnight's treatment, the dying man was up, dressed, and going about, to the pleasure and happiness of all concerned. Suggestion say some, purely imagination declare others, while "coincidence" and "expectancy" are called in to explain the foregoing by some and "fudge" will be the opinion of the learned (?) sceptical and egotistic. By all means, if "coincidence" or "imagination" can do so much good, it is a pity that it is not more frequently tried. The patient was satisfied, the friends pleased, and I -earned and received a handsome fee. I might here state this gentleman did not believe in Mesmerism— was rather opposed to the idea. I was not called until he was informed by his medical adviser "they could do nothing more for him." It was only a question of a few more days—the end. It was only by the persuasion of his friends that he was willing to try Mesmerism. Notwithstanding his personal objection to it, and his want of faith therein the work was done. Disease, in this case, furnished the physical and mental conditions of receptivity to the *influence* which in ordinary circumstances might otherwise have been rejected.

Men have successfully magnetised, controlled, and fascinated wild beasts. The eyes of man has arrested the approach of a lion, and caused him to retreat from the pursuit of prey; while beasts of prey have been known to fascinate and control their victims, whether birds, beasts, or human beings. Words which may be spoken with equal intelligence. feeling, and interest by two speakers, from the one speaker their effect is pleasing and attractive, but from the other—the *influence is magnetic—*

transfixes, infatuates, propels, and impels the life and actions of those who hear and see.

This influence is exercised by statesmen, generals, dictators, preachers, and musicians—by all who sway and govern the masses by the Influence of presence and voice—they who weave a potent spell about those who heat them. This force is a vital principle dependent on organisation, and may in a measure be cultivated or neglected—exercised knowingly or otherwise, and used for good or ill.

HOW THE MESMERIC POWER MAY BE CULTIVATED.

All persons can mesmerise some one. All persons can be mesmerised by some one. Many of the percentages, like some of the theories laid down by specialists, while containing some element of truth, are largely fanciful. Persons whom I could not mesmerise, might very successfully be operated upon by some other experimenter. Again, there are some who, having resisted all influence for many sittings, succumb in the end. There are predispositions which are positive in their nature—both physical and mental—which are not favourable to immediate, or any results. There are other temperaments and dispositions of such a mellow and negative character who would not, as a rule, make successful mesmerists —at least experimental mesmerists. It is also true, some are naturally more qualified to be successful mesmerists and healers than others. They are "gifted" having the mesmeric adaptability, just as others may be more poetical or musical. Exercise improves power, while non-exercise or excessive exercise deteriorates or exhausts it. *The Legitimate use of the power increases it*, while the loss of power may less seldom be attributed to its use than to other causes which may undermine the health and influence of the magnetiser.

Whatever contributes to the health, vitality, goodness of heart, and soundness of head of the mesmerist, contribute to his mesmeric power. Health and vitality being the leading requisites. The health habits of a mesmerist should be good, his will strong, while patience, endurance, perseverance, and sympathies should be marked features in his character. He should have a good, full, clear eye—colour not so much a. matter of importance, although persons of dark and hazel eyes make the most successful experimenters and entertainers, and those of dark blue, blue, and violet eyes, successful healers. A steady gaze is essential. No one can hope to be a mesmerist who cannot look another man or woman straight in the face. Further, a mesmerist should be able to make all necessary movements with ease and grace — "natural like." I have seen some good souls, possessing a fair aptitude for Mesmerism, so awkward in their movements as to arouse the visible in those upon whom they would operate. Nothing so keenly arouses the mind to resistance as the sense of ludicrous on the one hand, or anger or empty scepticism on the other. *Health* is largely a question of constitution—it is inbred—"comes by Nature." Its maintenance is requisite, but *the how* of its preservation and maintenance need not be entered upon here. Every mesmerist's life should be governed by "temperance in all things." He should abstain from gross foods, impure drinks, habits, and associations; cultivate the good and the true within himself. I might say that early and regular habits—morning bath, simple diet, adequate physical exercise, calm. ness or evenness of mind, will largely contribute to successful results. *Next to health*, comes self-government and the development of will, and the power to concentrate his energies. Will can be cultivated to a certain extent, but the initial power of will depend upon the phrenological development. A person deficient in Firmness, Self-Esteem, Conscientiousness, and Continuity is not likely to have a strong will. But if, in addition to the foregoing, they have those faculties which tend to timidity, lack of concentration, want of courage, as far as will is concerned, they would not make mesmerists at all.

The means used by Mesmerists for directing mesmeric influence are "the gaze"; by "passes," which are made "in contact"; and "at distance," and are "local" in character or "general"; by "breathing or blowing." Now these can be *easily* cultivated. In cultivating them it must be remembered they are not only the pantomime language of the *will* but that they are vehicles to convey something from the operator to the subject. At least let the mesmeriser act as if such were the case.

To cultivate "the gaze," the best time is in the morning, when the brain is raster, the mind dear and refreshed, and all the energies alive and wide awake. When a person is wearied or exhausted, the attempt to cultivate the gaze would probably end in sleep—Auto-Mesmerism or Hypnotism. In conversation, looking at the person quietly and steadily to whom you are speaking is a good plan; don't stare,, look straight into their eyes. *Think* your thoughts as well as *speak* them. There is not anything which will disconcert a courteous or discourteous liar than a *steady look*. In mesmerism you look with a purpose—your looks are to convey your intention, and will. The wandering eye—the blinking, winking, and irresolute eye—never accomplished much good in this world, mesmerically or any other way. When looking with a steady and quite gaze, *think,* picture to your mind a scene, incident phrase, or sentence. Should the person looked at give expression to the ideas or words induced by you repeat the process, again and again as opportunity is afforded, until you have eliminated the elements of accident and coincident.

While there is some element of thought-transference connected with this, you must first gain the power of looking naturally and steadily at a person or an object for a considerable length of time without weariness or fear of being hypnotised. Place a small piece of white paper on the centre of a looking-glass (a trying ordeal), and see how long you can look at it and the object behind it without winking or weariness. Repeat this again and again until you can look steadily at the object for ten and then for 15 minutes. Again in taking exercise, or if out for a long walk, take in some *object* at a distance which will take you some time to reach; while walking toward the object, gaze steadily at it as long as you can without impairing vision, causing weariness to the eyes, winking, or tears to flow, as in weeping. The habit of steady gazing can be cultivated in many ways. The most trying is to look at a bright light—a jet of gas or lime-light—for a certain period, and in unweariness such a way as to cultivate the physical assurance of or inferiority when looking at a human being. Any sign of weakness, such as inability to look at a person, about to be mesmerised steadily and for a length of time, would be prejudicial to successful results. The eyes should indicate strength of purpose, and show no sign of weakness. For this the optic nerve and the muscles of the eyes and eyelids must be educated for their work.

Having gone so far in the cultivation of the *gaze*, commence to use to some purpose. If at a place of amusement or at a lecture, sitting behind someone, look steadily at the nape of the neck, with the intention of giving them a desire to turn round. This can be done by persevering practice—a small percentage of successes will soon show you what can be done. You will begin to realise that the conscious direction of will by the eye becomes a most subtle and powerful mode or vehicle of thought.

The mesmerist must be powerful, and his subjects very sensitive receptive, and well educated, before the operations of will wholly and solely, are to be depended upon. It is not only right to cultivate the will but the means whereby it may be best expressed or conveyed.

Having cultivated the *gaze*, learn to make the passes, A little practice is necessary. All passes should be made quietly, easily, and gracefully, and in some respects with all the naturalness and kindliness with which a mother would pet a babe, or a good nurse soothe the pains of a sick person. At the same time, all passes should be made *with purpose*— not with great physical, but always with great mental action.

Passes are made long or general— from head to feet—and short or local — *i.e.,* directed to some region. They are also made, "at distans" or "in contact," whether local or general in character. The passes should be practised, so that they can be performed from half an hour to an hour and even longer, without apparently any physical weakness. Grace of physical action and strength of body are indicative of health, vigor, and will-power. These qualities can be cultivated. Practice is necessary to prevent weariness in making passes. A good plan for exercise might be adopted as follows: —Place a chair in the centre of a room (lock the door and proceed unobserved to the work), imagine a person seated on the chair, and take your stand opposite it for the purpose of putting him to sleep. Commence by making long passes. The hands, with fingers extended and directed toward the eyes of the supposed subject should then be lowered (at a distance of 2 to 5 inches) gradually and naturally down to his feet—that is making the downward or magnetic pass. The hands have now to be raised so as to resume original position. They should not be raised up in front of the patient's body, but on each side of him. The downward pass is to soothe, or produce sleep; the upward pass, as above described, is to enable you to repeat frequently the downward pass without undoing its work. In actual practice, mind-energy, or its concentration and *desired expression*, is put into your downward pass. No *intention* or concentration of mind is put into the upward pass; at the same time, it is also as well to keep it clear of the body, to prevent that disturbance which accidental reverse passes sometimes make. Downward passes — *i.e.*, from the head or brain to the feet or extremities — soothe or contribute to sleep; upward passes, to wakefulness. *Upward passes, with or without intention, never produce sleep.* It is thus deemed advisable to produce the upward pass in the way mentioned—not in front of, but dear and outside of the body of the subject.

Local passes, and "In contact" or touching the body, belong more particularly to the curative branch of the subject, and are used more frequently when there is no intention to produce sleep, but to cure disease. Of course, short passes can be and are made locally without contact for the same purpose. Sleep is often produced by local passes confined to the head, chest, arms, and sometimes terminating at the hypochondrium, or pit of the stomach. Passes can be and are made in every direction. The DOWNWARD PASSES INVARLABLY PRODUCE sleep.

Having made yourself at home by the cultivation of the gaze and the making of passes, you must learn how to breathe mesmerically. Certain wise physicians cured disease by "stroking" passes—and by "blowing" or breathing. Now there is an art in breathing as well as in *gaze* or in the *passes*. It can be cultivated. The method I suggest like all my methods, is natural and healthy—of great benefit to the individual, even though he never mesmerised any one. Each morning on rising, and at the earliest period of the day when fresh air can be obtained, the mesmeric adept should stand erect, with chest wen thrown out, mouth shut, and inhale slowly through his nostrils, and fully expand his lungs. It may be several weeks before he can take good long breaths and retain them, say, one minute in the lungs before exhaling. He should not exhale rapidly—on the contrary, exercise as much control over the last act as the former two, namely, the inspiration of the air and the power of retaining it in the lungs.

Having so far acquired power in this direction, the next is to know how to use it. Breathing can be used in several ways. Hot breathing, or air expired from the chest, is soothing, healing, curative. Cold breathing or the air blown slowly and deliberately from the compressed lips, has most salutary effects, and is arousing and wakeful in character. Some remarkable effects are obtained by breathing through flannel or clothing.

The cultivation of the steady eye, the graceful pass, the long and powerful breath, develop the health, the physical and mental powers. They help to strengthen and concentrate the will. The mesmeric influence is only valuable as it proceeds from a sound body and is directed by a sound mind. The foregoing simple processes are directed mainly to achieve that end.

CHAPTER V. HOW TO MESMERISE.

It is generally believed that only weak-minded soft, and hysterical persons can be successfully mesmerised—that persons of robust health, will, and character cannot be so affected. There never was a greater mistake. Reichenbach for many years selected his sensitives from delicate and hysterical persons while pursuing investigations into odylic force. He however, soon discovered his error, and found that healthy men and women made the best sensitives for investigation. Dr. Braid fell into the same error.

Charcot and others, including the whole range of recent hypnotists, have revived this error. The experience of all mesmerists—past and present — worthy of the name is this; the healthier and finer the organisation, the more perfect and exalted the manifestations.

There are relative conditions of superiority and inferiority in mesmerists and sensitives only. I have mesmerised men who were my superiors in every way —health, strength of body and mind— the only conditions of difference consisting of this important fact, that for the time being they approached the subject of Mesmerism with open minds—a desire to get at truth—and sat down with a non-resistant attitude of mind, perfectly willing to be mesmerised, and to record their own symptoms in connection -herewith, if possible. In the majority of cases the seventh or eighth sitting suffices to overcome all difficulties, and induce sleep in the most healthy and vigorous. There have, however, been exceptions to this. Don't waste time with a man who makes a bet through pride vanity, or ignorance, that he can't be mesmerised. Don't waste health and energy trying to influence him just then. His manner and words indicate that he will arouse ah his faculties to resist you presenting thereby positive and antagonistic mental conditions for

71

you to overcome. Men have done this. If you really want to mesmerise them then best plan is to throw them off their guard as to your intentions. But as soon as their opposition is cooled down a little, proceed *gently* and *steadily to impress them* with what Mesmerism has done and can do. Thus gradually and surely psychologise them, leading up to and preparing them for the final *coup.* In the end it may not be so difficult to mesmerise them as they at first imagined. The persistent man of business, the advocate of certain views—temperance, anti-slavery or what not,—the man with "a mission," the doctor of medicine, preacher, and lover, all adopt this method more or less unconsciously, because naturally, the mesmerist detecting the law, applies it consciously—that is all.

In natural sleep the heart beats slower, the pulses are calmer, there is less blood in the brain than in the waking state. By mesmeric processes you endeavour to bring about a similar psychological condition—every magnetic pass determining the result by retarding the flow of arterial blood to the brain. Also in natural sleep the eyes are turned upward and inward. A brief explanation of the muscles of the eye, and how they influence its movements, will be interesting. There are two sets of muscles. The superior, or oblique muscles, are involuntary in their action, and therefore are not subject to the action of the will. The inferior or straight muscles (of which there are four) are attached at ordinal points to the eye ball, and by their combined action the eyes are moved in every direction required for vision. The latter muscles are voluntary—that is, subject to the will of the individual. Now, when the eyes are withdrawn from the operations of the will, they are controlled involuntarily by the oblique muscles, and turned upward and inward. For Instance, in intense joy, in devotion, pain, sorrow, exhaustion, or bodily weakness, the eyes are turned up. This arises from the fact that the straight muscles resign their action, and the oblique muscles operate in their stead, and the eye is rolled upward under the eyelid. In acknowledging the presence of a superior and in the act of blowing, the eyes are "lifted up." See a girl in happy thought pondering on the future, a patient suffering from extreme pain, the devotee at worship be he idolater or Christian, or the wearied one waiting for transition to other and happier scenes on high—the same characteristic is observed. Thus, in sleep, in fainting, or in approaching death, the phenomenon is observed in all. The voluntary muscles resign their actions, insensibility prevails, the retina loses expression, and the pupil is turned up as described. Whatever contributes to this result contributes to sleep. The mesmeric operator avails himself of this and the foregoing in his endeavour to induce artificial sleep.

Hypnotists deliberately weary the inferior muscles of the eyes, trusting to automatic inhibition of the nerve centres for the result desired. Success in certain directions indicates they are not far astray. The mesmerist standing above his patient, or sitting in a chair a little higher up than the patient, unconsciously leads to the same automatic effect, but much more naturally. The hypnotist will cause the subject to strain his eyes at an object. The mesmerist desires his sensitive to be seated comfortably to look at him (the mesmerist), and if the sensitive or patient feel inclined to dose his eyes, to do so, or to sleep, to do so—the latter process being ore in. harmony with nature than the former.

HOW TO INDUCE SLEEP

Make your patient feel at home, disabuse his mind of fear, doubt, anxiety, and scepticism. (Mesmerise no one without the presence of some interested in the patient's welfare—parents, relatives, guardians, or medical adviser). Remove, if possible, all elements which are likely to arouse or excite the patient's mind. To succeed, the patient must either be naturally sensitive of your *influence*—i.e., passive and receptive—or he must be made so.

J. Coates, PHD.

Everything you do must tend to that condition. By action and speech—in everything you must show you know fully what you are about; there must be no timidity, hesitancy, or half-heartedness exhibited in your manner. You must create the instinctive feeling in the mind of your patient, "that is a man I can trust; that man or person will do me good" *and you will do it.* You can proceed to mesmerise by any of the processes, already recorded, or you can adopt this method, *viz,* —Let your patient be comfortably placed or seated; sit or stand before him, or just at his side. Ask him to pay no attention to his friends or surroundings, but resign himself to your care. He can either close his eyes, or look into yours. Inform him if he feels any strange or peculiar feelings—a sinking sensation, darkness of vision, nervous tremulousness, drowsiness or an inclination to sleep, not to resist but give way. It will be all right, and you will see him through.

Next, for five minutes or so, take hold of his hands in an easy, comfortable manner, or he can place his hands upon his knees, and you can lay yours with a just perceptible physical pressure on the top of them. Remain thus in contact until there is no apparent difference in temperature between your hands and his. Direct your eyes to his, or, rather, to the organ of "Individuality," or that portion of the head just situated between the two eyebrows, at the root of the nose. Exercise your *will* calmly and steadfastly towards the desired end—sleep. Gradually remove your hands from his, and place them on his head for two or three minutes, covering his forehead at each temple with the hollow of your hand, With fingers resting on head and your thumbs converging towards "Individuality,"—Slight pressure with the hands on the temples is desirable, as it tends to check the inflow of blood to the head per the temporal arteries. You will now proceed to further *charge* the brain with your influence by passes directed to that end, always downward over the head and face—forehead, tophead, sidehead, and backhead —all coming under your direction, so far as such

74

passes can be made with *direct intent* and with ease and comfort. You will also facilitate our purpose by pointing the tips of your fingers toward the eyes and temples, but throughout there must be neither vulgar staring nor thumb pressure. You will continue making these movements until the eye-lids tremble, become heavy, or close. In some cases it is advisable to close the eyelids and fasten them by downward passes, and thus hasten the result desired. When I say hasten the result — *viz.* the mesmeric sleep of the person operated on— do not mean the mesmerist to hasten: *he should never be in a hurry.* When the patient has exhibited the signs mentioned, you now proceed with both local and by general passes at *distance* to abstract your influence (but not to awaken your now-sensitive) by moving your hands with fingers extended slowly from his head to his fingers, both inside and outside the arms, also from the forehead down in front of the body to pit of stomach, and then towards the knees. At the termination of each pass raise the hands (as described in practising the passes) and commence again. Continue these passes for some time after he or she has apparently fallen asleep.

If you do not succeed at first, proceed at subsequent sittings as if you had no previous failure; and when once you succeed in putting a person asleep your power to do so will be enhanced, and your future percentages will increase in due proportion. When you have obtained satisfactory evidence of sleep, it is advisable to try no experiments for the first two or three sittings, beyond the following. Let the patient sleep on for some time, and then quietly wake him up. *Don't do it suddenly.* You might spoil for ever a good subject by so doing. Stand behind or before your sensitive, and make slowly and then briskly upward passes (palms of the hands up) in *front of the face* and blow steadily on the forehead, when your patient will awake much surprised and benefitted by the sleep. With a little more experience you can arrange with your patient when he will awake of his own accord. When this is done, the sensitive will always awake at the time arranged. This arrangement or experiment is capable of considerable extension or modification.

HOW TO CULTIVATE CLAIRVOYANCE
OR CLEAR SIGHT.

Hypnotic and platform subjects do not make clairvoyants. *Clairvoyance* can only be cultivated by proceeding in the first instance as above. I may add here *clairvoyance* is a reality. Its existence in various subjects has been proved again and again, and has been testified to by so many credible witnesses, past and present, at home and abroad. To put it briefly, it is either an exhibition of gross ignorance or gross impertinence and ignorance, to deny the existence of the phenomenon. Sensitives have foretold illness, death, and the recovery of patients, prescribed remedies for disease, traced stolen and strayed property. *Introvision or prevision*, have been and are phenomena so common in the experience of mesmerists of the old school, and so amply recorded, that I need but briefly refer to them here. The mesmeriser recognises that in order to act upon a patient, there must be a connecting link of sympathy between them. This connecting link is not a creation of suggestion and ignorance by which the phantasies and illusions of hypnotic patients are created, but a real link by which (moral, mental, and physical) sympathy is thoroughly established between the mesmeriser on the one hand and his sensitive on the other. By concentration of the will and the use of the means, the *rapport* or *sympathy* desired between the operator and the patient is effected; the honest desire to relieve pain and cure disease then finds a ready channel of communication. If in some instances the action for good is intensified by faith in the patient, it is only natural it should be so.

That *clairvoyance* can be induced by Mesmerism is not to be doubted. The mesmeriser and his sensitive are distinct entities, *egos*—individuals, if you will —both having their respective organisation, temperament, and character. The primary action of Mesmerism should be that of spirit acting on spirit, mind on mind—such action being that of direction, or education, and sympathy. Secondly, the action of Mesmerism is that of spirit or mind over organisation. Therefore we have the mind of the mesmeriser influencing the mind of the sensitive directly, or through the organisation indirectly. Mesmeric operations in their highest and truest character are spiritual, then mental, then physical Hypnotic experiments are physical first, mental afterward, spiritual seldom. *Clairvoyance* is possible in Mesmerism, impossible in the latter. Clairvoyance— "clear seeing"—might be called "soul-sight," as a vivid ray of electric light flashed suddenly out into midnight darkness reveals much that is hidden with sudden and startling clearance. So it happens in Mesmerism; when the senses are completely subdued; the passions and the emotions allayed by the mesmerist, then the subtle powers of the spirit (pneuma) and the spirit body (psyche) shine forth and reveal the hidden mysteries of mind.

Mere physical mesmerists, "electro biologists," and hypnotists, although they can cure disease, and have induced many strange and peculiar phenomena, in certain classes of subjects, they do not subdue the physical in the foregoing sense, and they cannot educe mental and psychical phenomena. The best clairvoyant sensitives have been women from about 15 to 25, whose organisations were healthy, refined and pure, and whose heads were favourably developed in the spiritual, moral, intuitive and mental faculties. The most successful developers of *clairvoyance* in such were those who believed in the reality of soul and things spiritual, and who instinctively looked for their expression and manifestation in their sensitives, but who did nothing more than subdue the physical or outward senses in the sensitive, and wisely left the development of *clairvoyance* to the progress of growth, carefully watching the avoidance of all weariness, mental and spiritual exhaustion, in those under their care. To develop *clairvoyance* in subjects there must be no "hot-house planting" or forcing about it or them. Caution to both mesmerists and sensitives: There must be no hurry. Mesmerists can furnish favourable conditions, but they cannot create *clairvoyance*.

With the foregoing explanatory digressions, I assume that your patient has been put asleep, and that you have been able not only to comfortably accomplish this, but to awaken him—(some fall into apparent sleep, or into a natural sleep. Should you address them, they will either awake or sleep on. Should they, however, answer your question—some simple question as "Do you feel comfortable?" in a quiet and intelligent way, the sensitives have, in all probability, passed into the mesmeric somnambulistic stage, which frequently precedes the lucid or clairvoyant stage). Having gained confidence, and satisfied yourself of your ability to proceed, you will learn two or three things—one, perhaps, the most surprising of all, *viz* , that he or she is not your subject in the sense in which the term is used—a sensitive, rather—who has a distinct and exalted individuality, of which you and he were not conscious before, in this state he will converse with you as a self-possessed, dear-headed, and far-seeing being, from whom you may learn something about yourself, your life conditions, how to improve them, about the powers of the human soul or spirit, and the destiny and well-being of the race here and hereafter, whether you are prepared to accept this or not will greatly depend upon your individual experience in such matters In reply to questions, which must not be *hastily*, or injudiciously, or suggestively put, you will ascertain what process of mesmerising agrees with your sensitive best; also, what modes of procedure to adopt to perfect his condition; how he wishes to sleep, and when he will awake, and when he should enter the condition, or state, again; what he feels, and what are his experiences in that state; whether he observes a *light* in his brain, the position and the character of it; whether he sees you, or perceives you, or in what degree he is in sympathy (or otherwise) with you as his mesmeriser; the kind and nature of his *power of vision*, if any, and the situation of the same in the forehead, crown of the head, or hypochondrium; also, what you can do to improve his lucidity, etc. In this way you will ascertain in time what powers he possesses, whether he can look into his own organisation, or yours, and that of others with whom you place him in contact—what he can *see* (*i.e* objects) or *discern* (*i.e.* things on a mental and spiritual plane); whether he can diagnose his own condition or that of others; also, if he can *travel*, visit places of interest to you, and describe the places and the people, or report to you what they do and say. So go on in your investigations patiently from day to day. Do not attempt anything in a hurry, or attempt to force results. You must always be kind and firm. Gently check what appears to you to be incongruous and establish the fullest confidence, sympathy, or rapport between yourself and sensitive. See how far he perceives your intentions, thoughts, or wishes —unexpressed by you. Be always ready, in any reasonable way, to improve his condition, especially in the further development of his spiritual, moral, and mental powers. Finally, if he should *see*, and converse with *unseen intelligence, disembodied human spirits*, do not hastily conclude that such is impossible. Be patient, take time and judge of the reality, or otherwise, of such contingency, however strange or *abnormal* it might appear by the *internal evidence conveyed* to you in the message, or communication made to you, by your sensitive. For this class of phenomena your sitting should be held at a regular hour daily, and terminated whenever your patient desires, or by mutual agreement, or whenever in your judgment it has lasted long enough. If following up the investigations daily, an hour would probably be long enough for each sitting. Male sensitives are best for scientific and business purposes—the very best subjects are the most difficult to get under control at first— females for literary, inspirational, and pre-visional experiments. I have found no difficulty in mesmerising persons of sanguine-nervous temperaments, and persons of all colours of hair and eyes, save black, dark brown, and hazel. Negroes and Hindoos are, however, very sensitive to mesmeric influence. My experience is confirmed by that of other leading mesmerists. It is worthy of remark that my temperament is not of the sanguine-nervous type, and that my influence is most effective, as a rule, over those who are completely contrasted from myself. Of course there are modifications of this, yet the rule appears to be that contrasts of temperament are favourable to mesmeric experiments, and that similarity of temperament is not. There is no reason why persons, otherwise healthy and sound, of strong will and genial sympathies, should not make good mesmerists, although they are of the sanguine nervous type, and belong to the auburn-haired and blue-eyed order of humanity. Yet for experiments, public work, strength of will and purpose, I have found the nervous and bilious form of temperament —that is the tail, dark, wiry type—the most effective.

HOW TO CULTIVATE PSYCHOMETRY.

Psychometry (soul-measuring) is allied to clairvoyance. Like it, or *second night*, it is often a normal possession. It can be cultivated in many who have never been mesmerised. Yet the best class of mesmeric sensitives always make good psychometrical mediums. As physiognomy and phrenology give us by external indications some knowledge of the character and dispositions of our fellows, psychometry gives a keener and deeper insight; it passes the boundary of the external, and *measures the soul.*

Intuition (manifested through the organ of Human Nature), has been called the sixth sense. Reason is a mathematician. With her, nothing must be taken for granted. She argues, demonstrates, and logically concludes. To prove the centre of a circle, she will approach her task with algebraic formula — square and compass. Not so with intuition. She will lay her finger on the spot, and say. "There it is," and she is right. *Psychometry* is intuition, exalted or spiritualised. Certain organisations are more favourable to its manifestations than others. 'Woman, for many reasons, makes a better psychometrical sensitive than man. Her brain is particularly adapted for its psychological expression. By Psychometry, true traits of character can be unfolded and traced to their basis in ancestry. The circumstances and relations of the forgotten in family history, at a stated period, can be brought to light by the *influence* still left on some old relic, trophy, gem, or piece of tapestry. There are authenticated instances of valuable mines having been discovered by it. It is a well-known historical fast fact that Mrs. Wm. Denton (wife of Professor Denton the celebrated geologist), discovered copper mines in Canada as well as gold mines in Austria, by means of her psychometrical gift. This lady was also a great help to her husband in his scientific investigations.

In some instances it has been employed in tracing crime, and in finding stolen and lost articles. While not prepared to advance so much in the favour of *Psychometry* as claimed for it by various authorities. I am inclined to give it a place here, as its cultivation in my opinion can do no harm, and may be a source of innocent amusement and instruction to many. To cultivate it the following modes may be adopted. Place your subject in the mesmeric deep, sufficiently deep to be entirely lost to the consciousness of external things. Give him a handkerchief, pocket-knife, watch or other much used article belonging to a third person whom you do not know, but whose appearance, character, disposition, can be vouched for subsequently by trusted parties. Tell your sensitive to relate what are his feelings, and what are the sensations (if any) which he experiences from the articles placed in his possession. If care has been taken and no suggestions, etc., made, it is more than likely the sensitive will give at first trial a broken description of general indications of the appearance and disposition of the party to whom the things belong. At subsequent sitting the power to diagnose surroundings, history, and character, will increase.

You can then intensify the conditions by getting the articles rolled up in paper by third parties in such a way that you do not know yourself what they are. Your sensitive's descriptions however faulty at first, will become correct in the main, then singularly accurate, then marvellously so. His keenness of spiritual perception will be so great as to go back to all the conditions which have surrounded the life of the person examined, from his childhood, and into the motives which have influenced certain departures, mistakes, and successes in his life. In time your sensitive on being presented an old key, or axe, or a geological specimen, will give you an equally accurate and reliable description of its history and associations, which will make you declare that truth is stronger than fiction. In some instances, without being put asleep, *simply sitting in a passive condition*, psychometry can be cultivated.

HOW TO DEVELOP THOUGHT READING.

To this category belong thought transference and mind-reading. The performances of Mr. Irving Bishop, Mr. Stuart Cumberland, and Mr. Edwin James, were called thought-reading entertainments. The entertainments of the two former being a compound of trickery very bad conjuring *muscle—reading nous*, and audacity, combined with effeminate organisations, furnished them with the requisite qualifications for their exhibition. Mr. Edwin James has a higher claim to the title of thought reader than either of the other two, because he really gave an excellent intellectual treat for an entertainment. Travesties of modem spiritualism, and conjuring in any form, are ignored by this gentleman. Of course he finds the pin, blindfolded, and reproduces much of the time and patience-killing experiments of the other two gentlemen. He is much superior to them in this. He disclaims being a thought-reader, and claims only to reproduce such thoughts to which a physical shape has been given. If three or four of his audience are formed into a striking group upon the platform representing a tragic, dramatic, or domestic scene, should his medium picture the incident well upon his mind, he (Mr. James) can reproduce the scene by replacing the aforesaid individuals exactly in a similar position that in which the committee had then previously. He accomplishes this by a twofold process, psychological impressions, and by muscle indications. His exhibition is the most genuine of the class. Thought-reading is necessarily in an elementary stage just now. Mesmeric subjects in the waking state, and young children who have not been mesmerised, make the best sensitives. The editor of the *Nineteenth Century* formulated an ingenious theory about twenty years ago in the *Spectator*, to account for the phenomenon. It is difficult to understand how scientific men can accept such a *theory of brain waves*, and a *universal unpalpable elastic ether* as an explanation of the admitted facts, that thought can be read and thought can be transferred, seeing that they reject the less difficult hypothesis of Zoo-Magnetism or nervous fluid—a material medium of surpassing and inconceivable tenuity. It is of less interest to many how it is done, as it is true? Professor Barrett, of the Royal College of Science, Dublin, who is also an indefatigable member of the society for Psychical Research, has perhaps more than any other man. In the United Kingdom devoted his energies to the scientific investigations of this subject. I select one of the cases on which he has reported, and which occurred at the house of the Rev. Creery of Burton, which will perhaps put in clearer light what thought-reading is, and how it is done, than any lengthy description of mine.

"Easter, 1881.—Present, Mr. and Mrs. Creery and family and Mr. F. Barrett, the narrator. One of the children was sent into an adjoining room, the door of which I saw was closed. On returning to the sitting-room and closing its door also, I thought upon some object in the house fixed upon at random. Writing the name down, I showed it to the family present, the strictest silence being preserved throughout. We then all silently thought of the name of the thing selected. In a few seconds the door of an adjoining room was heard to open, and after a very short interval the child would enter the sitting-room, generally speaking, with the object selected. No one was allowed to leave the sitting-room after the object had been fixed upon, and no communication with the child was conceivable as her place was often changed. Further, the only instructions given to the child were to fetch some object in the house that I would fix upon and together with the family silently keep in mind, to the exclusion as far as possible of all other ideas. In this way I wrote down, among other things, a hair-brush—it was brought; an orange —it was brought; a wine-glass—it was brought; an apple—it was brought; a toasting fork—failed on the first attempt, a pair of tongs being brought, but on a second trial it was brought. With another child, a cup was written down by me— it was brought; a saucer—this was a failure, a plate being brought. No second trial allowed. The child being told it was a saucer, replied. "That came into my head but I hesitated, as I thought it unlikely you would name a saucer after a cup had been brought."

Altogether, 382 trials were made in the course of six days. Professor Barrett continues— "Once most stoking piece of success, when the things selected was divulged to none of the family, was five cards running named correctly on the first {rial—

the odds against this happening once in our series being considerably over one million to one. We had altogether a good many similar batches, the two longest runs being eight consecutive successes, once with cards and once with names, where the adverse odds in the former case were over 142 millions to 1, and, in the latter, something, incalculably greater. Walls and closed doors made no difference.

"The willing game" is too well-known to find extended notice here. But it makes a pleasant and easy introduction to thought-reading experiments and to Mesmerism as a drawing-room entertainment among friends. Thought-reading can also be tested in this way. Send one of the company out of the room, then hide an article upon which all the rest have agreed, in a place also agreed upon. When the person selected enters the room, let all be silent, each person present thinking of the article and where it is hidden. It is more than likely if the searcher acts upon his first impression entering the room, he or she will find the article. This can be improved upon by thinking of a word—such as "hope," "faith," "father," "mother," "good," etc. By acting on the first inspiration, the medium selected may utter the exact word, or the company may decide on a written symbol or simple design. The most magnetic person in the room should then be selected to convey the impression to the sensitives, and so on, as good sensitives are discovered. By magnetic I mean the most positive and most successful person in the party in impressing or influencing others.

CHAPTER VI. CURATIVE MESMERISM.

The powers of the early Christians, whether natural "gifts of healing," or both, were intensified by the simplicity and purity of their living, and the reality of their faith. They doubted not, yet where they doubted they could do no miracles. The man who has "no heart," to relieve disease, or, having sympathy, has no will to do so, is either without the power to do good, or doubting his power, is unable to use it. From such no "virtue" can go forth to heal. Where there is sympathy for suffering, the desire to relieve or remove it, and the *will* to do so, the way soon opens up, and the suffering is removed.

The most powerful healers I ever came in contact with had strong, healthy vital organisations, and were large-hearted, kindly-disposed persons. The fact is, that persons with devitalised organisations do not make magnetic healers. They cannot give what they have not got, A bankrupt should not bestow gifts—a pauper cannot give alms.

In hydropathy, *manipulations* continue a large part of the treatment. Great benefits are done if the bathmen or women—the shampooers—are healthy, cheerful, and buoyant people.

The success which attends certain wonderful embrocations (which are often nothing more than simple and innocuous oils and newspaper puffs) may be traced to the faithful carrying out of the direction —"Rub in briskly with a warm hand for several minutes." External remedies possessing valuable properties are always rendered more efficacious by the observance of such directions.

The *healing gift* is more or less enjoyed by all persons. The large hearted and intuitive physician, the mother, nurse, or friend, whose presence is more enjoyed, and whose advice is most desired by the sick, win have the gift in a large degree. Such gift, when exercised by goodness and sympathy, must ever have a *wholesome* and healing effect.

The weak, tender, and delicate, when the heart and head work together, can accomplish much, however. The tired mother, wearied with nursing, does not lose her charm to soothe. Gentle and tender, ever more thoughtful of others than herself, her diligent hands, bring peace and blessing with them at all times. Her little boy, running from her side, a moment or two to play, falls and cuts himself; his little knees are all crushed and bruised by the stones on the roadway. She lifts the child upon her knee, pets and rubs his knees *with her hands*, gently and sympathetically. She is only petting him and rubbing the dirt off, you say; she is doing more—she is throwing her love and *life force* into every touch with the result *that the bleeding ceases, and the pain is gone.* Here the mother, without thought of mesmeric or hypnotic speculations, obeys her maternal instincts, and thus intuitively exercises "the gift of healing." Herein lies the secret of *Curative Mesmerism*, with this difference: the mesmerist consciously and determinately exercises his powers, seeking to accomplish by tried and approved methods what the other, in a lesser degree, had brought about intuitively.

Although delicate and sensitive females, from their sympathetic and patient natures, have been very successful in the treatment of disease—at considerable loss to themselves, however—no one should undertake to treat disease of a severe character unless they have abundance of health and vitality; and have also the determination, patience, and sympathy requisite to make them good healers. Ladies make excellent healers, just as they make the best nurses. The *gift* can be readily cultivated by them, and by practice put to good use. For many reasons woman would be the best magnetiser for woman, man for a man, husband for wife, (wife for husband, and father and mother for children etc.; but this cannot always be. There is no reason why the professional healer, male and female, should not be trusted and esteemed as honourable in their work and position as the physician or minister.

"Covet the best gifts" is the advice of one sacred writer. To my mind, the power to heal disease is the gift of gifts, the one most to be desired by the mesmeric aspirant. All other phenomena educed or evolved by the mesmeric process, however startling or interesting are valueless unless they contribute to the requirements of the healing art.

Dr. Hitchman, M.R.C.S., Eng. (formerly of Guy's Hospital, London, late of Leeds Cancer Hospital, and of Liverpool), many years ago informed me "that it was erroneous to suppose that Mesmerism was only beneficial in nervous diseases. He had seen it arrest the progress and finally cure cancer," and I know, from personal experience, that diseases other than those for which it has been most frequently used. I have known it to reduce colds, to allay inflammatory symptoms, and to cure billious attacks, to reduce *white swelling*, a painful disease of the knee joints and equally to relieve the agony arising from a cut or crushed finger or limb.

Many of these cases were undertaken under medical supervision, while others, the larger number, were those which came to me in the course of professional work, either attracted by lectures, or recommended by the friends of those who had at some previous time received some benefit from Mesmerism. Although I cannot record the cure of cancer, like Dr. Illiotson or Dr. Hitchman, or absolute cures of total blindness like Dr. Mack, my pretty wide and general experience enables me to declare my undoubted conviction, that there is scarcely any form of disease which may not be at least relieved where not cured, by the steady, persevering, and judicious use of the mesmeric processes.

Massage, shampooing, muscular and kinetic movements, are but different modes of local mesmeric treatment. These terms are more fashionable in some quarters than the word Mesmerism—that is of little consequence, if good is done.

Some years ago, I applied local Mesmerism to the cure of "writer's cramp," and ailments of that class, with great success. The manipulations and directions seemed to cure the most obstinate cases. Personally, I attributed the success to Animal Magnetism; but not a few medical men attributed the success to deftness of direction and power of manipulation, which might be termed "tactus eruditus," in plain English "knock." There is no secret about it and yet I admit it is not easily taught. My processes might be called "massage, combined with local gymnastics."

Persons suffering from disease—disease not merely confined to or classed as nervous derangements —are particularly susceptible to Mesmerism. Apart from the desire, if any, of the patients for relief or cure the departure from the normal state—health — renders them specially receptive to the influence of a healthy operator. Many persons who in a state of health have, been opposed to Mesmerism, or incredulous concerning its power, have been among the first to seek from it the comfort of its curative influence which at other times they would have repelled.

CURATIVE PROCESSES.

The mesmeric processes adopted in the cure of diseases are those of sleep, and when it is necessary the application of remedies suggested by the sensitive in sleep, or by your clairvoyant, in the case of one for another patient. In such cases, medicines may be ordered, baths prescribed, rules of diet pointed out, or certain processes of treatment ordered. And you will, if satisfied with the *bondfides* of your sensitive's powers of diagnosis and general lucidity, faithfully carry them out, The mesmeric treatment for the cure of disease may be purely local or general in character, exercised solely with the intention to alleviate and cure disease, without producing sleep, sleep not being necessary in the majority of cases. If necessary, you know how to bring it about. Nothing is worth doing that is not worth doing well. If you want to cure disease set about it, and "whatever *your hands* find to do, do it with all your might," *i.e.* put your *soul* into it. Avoid ail experiments and direct your attention, energies, and, in fact, all your powers, to the work—the most needed work — the cure of your patient.

By disease, or dis-ease, we find a disturbance of the *life forces*, and want of harmony or ease throughout the whole organisation, corresponding to a want of equable temperature, such as a hot aching head with cold feet, a cold stomach, and correspondingly defective digestion, a heated front head with mental excitement, a heated backhead with temper, or diseased amatory desires, etc. By local and general passes, according to the circumstances, in each case you will dissipate the heated or feverish symptoms banish all evil influences, and infuse warmth and life where there are none. Equalise the "magnetic circulation" throughout the organisation by withdrawing from each organ, or part, as are overcharged, and conveying the same to those parts where there is feebleness or deficiency, and finally, imparting such magnetism from yourself as you are willing and able to give to restore them to a state of case or health again.

Remember, Mesmerism is not a cure-all. There are diseases of such a character, arising from hereditary taint, constitutional defects, and organic causes, which can never be cured in this world, only you, as a mesmerist, should not say so. Give help when and where you can, according to your strength. So that in these, medically and humanely speaking, utterly hopeless and intractable cases you are not to refuse aid, seeing there are few cases where the mesmeric influence will not soothe and relieve pain, quiet the nervous system, restore sleep and strength in a large measure, and, what is not to be despised, impart a cheerful and hopeful spirit to the patient.

In chronic and acute diseases, especially when there is a periodicity in attack, sleep is recommended to break that periodicity, and to lengthen the intervals between attacks. In all mental, psychological, and highly nervous troubles sleep is advised. When this is necessary, mesmerise by the long pass from head to feet; the patient being in bed, or lying upon the sofa, will materially facilitate your operations. You will soon begin to see the effects of your attendance by the improvement in your patient. When the patient "looks for you," is impatient for your visit, and wearies for the next, it is not a bad sign; it indicates your influence and presence to be refreshing and restorative in character. Good doctors and nurses have the same characteristics. If your presence or influence is in any way disagreeable to your patient, and upon the third or fourth visit you are satisfied of this, give up the treatment. You can do no good, although another may. But do not give up a case simply because favourable results are tardy m making their appearance. Where your influence is not disagreeable, it is your duty to persevere and hope for the best. You cannot do harm, and you may do great good.

When there is nervousness and great debility, operate from the head—back-head—downward, long passes at first, and then short passes locally. If the action of the heat is weak or palpitation is characteristic, breathe in upon it at the termination of each treatment. You will be surprised at the warmth and generous feeling transferred throughout your patient's organism in consequence. You can subdue the most violent coughing fit by steadily, and gently breathing upon the spine, just between the shoulder-blades of your patient—child or adult. So long as the clothing, under or upper, is not made of silk, the breathing will be effectual. The lungs should be fully expanded, the mouth placed dose to the part, as near as the clothing will admit, and a steady, strong stream of breath thrown in upon the place. The moment the mouth is removed, the open hand should be placed over the place while filling the lungs to repeat the operation, which may be done several times.

In rheumatic and neuralgic derangements and ailments of that class, and in cuttings, bruises, and bums, the treatment is often purely local—the passes following the course of the nerves of sensation. *In mesmeric treatment it is just as well to remember there is no need, to remove the clothing under any circumstances*, unless it is composed of silk or other non-conducting material. *For economical reasons old clothing is better than new.*

Toothache is a common affliction. You will have many opportunities of immediately relieving it, if not effectually and ultimately curing it. A very good and practical method of cure is to lay your hand upon the affected side of the face, and hold it there for a few minutes, and this prepares the face for the next movement. Then place a piece of flannel over the ear (on the same side of the head as the toothache); keep your hand still on the face, but now over the flannel, with the other hand over the head, holding the upper portion of the flannel (or fourfold ordinary pocket handkerchief) over the ear. Now breathe strongly and steadily into the ear through the covering thus made. Do this two or three times strongly willing the removal of the pain. A warm, soothing influence will reach the offending tooth, and peace will ensue. At the last breath remove, the handkerchief quickly, and the pain will be gone. A little success in this direction will enable you to your hand at more serious business.

Violent headaches—even arising from billious attacks—can be relieved in a remarkable way by *passes*. Stand behind the patient, who should be seated. Place your hands on the forehead. Keep them there a little, and then make short *passes in contact* gently and firmly, with slight pressure on the temples and backward over the side and top head to the crown; then draw out, and shake your finger as if you were throwing water off them, and proceed again to make passes as before. In five to fifteen minutes relief will be given, if the pain is not removed altogether.

In rheumatism and such diseases, in which pain is a marked characteristic, Mesmerism "works like a charm." The patient is always pleased to be relieved of pain, and as the pain subsides, his mental and physical conditions become more favourably receptive to your *influence*. If, in treating a rheumatic patient, a pain is moved—say from the shoulder to the middle of the arm above the elbow—continue your treatment, and. instead of drawing passes to the fingers, endeavour to draw the pain down to and out of, the elbow joints. If you are able to move the pain, if only an inch from its original position, you have control over it, and it will be able, in due course, to remove it altogether.

MESMERISED WATER AND ITS VIRTUES.

Mesmerised water is a most powerful remedial agent. It can be taken internally as a medicine or a drink, or used externally by compress or in a bath. The value of mesmerised water is best judged by the results produced by it. I have known the most obstinate cases of constipation to have been effectually cured by it—some of the patients having for years found it necessary to take a pill or some other strong aperient every second day to make the bowels act; and in one case of a poor man, in whom the peristaltic action of the bowels seemed to be temporarily paralysed, who remained without action for a fortnight. Drugs were used freely: without effect. He was given a glassful of mesmeric water but twice, when his difficulty was remedied. The treatment was continued for five weeks, and he was completely restored. In this case I never even saw the patient. The mesmerised water was sent from Liverpool, and administered by a friend to the patient in Blackburn.

I value mesmerised water because by its use you get at the organisation therapeutically in the absence of personal magnetisation or attendance. The water in a short time will get into the circulation, and wherever there are nerves and arteries your curative life force will be carried on its healing mission. You will find similar astonishing results from the use of magnetised mediums such as flannels, paper, and pillules. Lay your hand upon a looking-glass for a few minutes then raise it—you will find a vaporous impression of your hand upon the glass, which will die away from perceptible vision in a short time, so that no one would think or imagine your hand had ever been there. Breathe upon the looking-glass at any subsequent time, three days or a week afterwards (providing the glass has not been thoroughly cleaned in the meantime), and by that breathing the last impression of your hand will come to sight again, as though it had always been there. So it often happens that, unseen to mortal eyes or hidden from perceptible vision, or beyond scientific or medical detection, we are always laying our hands upon, and creating influences on and about our fellows, which only need the opportunity or right breathing to expose or reveal the past actions and thoughts so forgotten. Thus you cannot speak, look, or shake hands with others without leaving your mark there. If this is true in the ordinary affairs of life, where no man can live or die to himself, how much more so is it with the mesmerist, who acts with *intention*? If he has any power at all, surely it will tell; and it does tell.

To mesmerise or magnetise water (See Chapter IV), hold the tumbler of water in your left hands, or if left-handed in your right hand, and hold the fingers of the other hand over it, pointing down towards the water; convey to it, by concentration of desire, your intentions; thus you may make it an aperient an astringent, a tonic, or a nervine. The ultimate idea is to soothe and tranquilise the system, and enable the *vis medicatrix nature* to do its work for the recovery of the patient.

Mesmerised water should be made of water carefully filtered—if possible, of spring water filtered—so as to form a natural, healthy, and pure drink, and thereby furnishing all the better vehicle for your *influence*. Such water cannot always conveniently be sent to a distance. In that case mesmerised pillules will be found useful. Hold the pure and innocuous sugar pillules in your hands, and roll them in the hollow of, or between your hands, and "breathe upon" them before bottling. I use the ordinary homoeopathic pillule, as it is before medication. Bandages or belts for the waist, soles, or socks, for the feet I have found of great service. Even the diet of the patient, as well as the water he drinks, can be imbued with this *communicable life-force* with benefit to the patient.

I do not think it possible to eliminate faith and suggestion from mesmeric operation *in toto*, certainly not as long as we are dealing with beings capable of exercising faith or being influenced by *suggestion*. Shall the preacher or the physician or the teacher cease their particular labours because these subtle forces act so powerfully with those with whom they have to do? I think not. Neither should the mesmerist.

J. Coates, PHD.

CONDITIONS OF CURE

I cannot leave this part of the subject—to me the most interesting and, I believe, the most important without pointing out some auxiliaries to this, the magnetic healing art.

There are certain conditions favourable to cure as there are certain conditions (almost) provocative of disease; on the latter we need not expressly dwell — dirt and impurity in surroundings and habits—overeating and drinking—lack of healthy useful, or suitable employment. A reckless or prodigal disposition unhealthy employments and poverty, certainly engender and disseminate disease. On the other hand, temperance and moderation in the individual, a cheerful, calm, and religious frame of mind, personal cleanliness and domestic sanitation and hygiene—healthy surroundings and suitable occupation or employment—promote and sustain health. Suppose a patient is cured of neuralgia or rheumatism, or some pulmonary affection of the lungs, or weakness of the heart, or gout by the aid of Mesmerism—accompanied by certain health conditions — such as moderation in eating or drinking, bathing, total abstinence from drugs—although the same were only alcohol and tobacco. This patient gathers strength and vitality and is pronounced cured. If in the course of a few months after cure, he were to relapse into old habits again, and his disease were to return, the result would not be surprising. On the contrary, nothing else could be expected, *seeing the conditions of cure had been neglected.* Mesmerism would not be to blame.

The mesmeric practitioner should endeavour to ascertain the cause of all diseases he is called upon to treat, and as far as lies within his power or direction, or within the ability of his patient labour to have the cause or causes removed.

All patients are better to be extremely moderate in diet, even in eating those things which they like, and which will agree with them the best. Fruit in due season, whole-meal bread milk, butter, eggs, lean beef, mutton, chicken, white fish etc., in *moderation*, form excellent articles of diet. "Pure food makes pure blood."

All patients are the better of a bath of some kind *daily*. The care of the skin is a most essential condition of cure. The morning bath—that is the bath taken immediately on rising—is most excellent. It should take the form of a rapid wash of the whole body—warm, tepid, or cold water, according to the health and vitality of the patient The process of renovation is largely carried on during sleep, and impurities are thrown out and collected upon the skin during the night. These are removed by the morning bath, purify the skin, and give favourable condition of cure to the organisation. This hygiene of the skin is useful in liver and kidney diseases, bladder, and urinary complaints. Much crankiness, nervous uneasiness, depression, lowness of spirits and actual disease, etc., can be traced to laziness and the want of personal cleanliness. A warm cleansing or a vapour bath in addition to the foregoing might be taken with advantage every week. A tepid bath once a day will be found useful in most cases. Time for taking— best in the afternoon.

Two or three meals a day or more; baths, how many or how few, must depend upon the peculiarities of each case. Fresh air, surroundings, and even companionship, are matters not to be overlooked by the mesmerist. If he has any influence at all over disease, he must have it over mind; and if over mind, it should be in a righteous and healthy direction.

If the case is taken under medical supervision, the duty of the mesmerist is to work steadily for the ultimate cure of the disease, leaving the medical and hygienic advice entirely in the hands of the medical practitioner. If you have any suggestion to make, any suspicions, doubts, communicate them to the doctor in charge— in fact, consult with him, and leave all the directions entirely in his hands. You will always find this course advisable. The medical adviser is pleased, being duly honoured, and the patient or friends are not perplexed by divided authority, and you will have free course to do the work to your satisfaction.

The medical man who consents to a mesmerist being called in to a case will, as a rule, be happy to second any reasonable proposition which the mesmerist may make.

CHAPTER VII. HOW TO GIVE AN ENTERTAINMENT.

Mesmerism, as an entertainment, either in drawing-room, or more publicly in platform exhibitions, is always fascinating. There is an air of the wonderful and mysterious about mesmeric entertainments which is always sure to draw the public. Where such exhibitions are judiciously and humanely given, the public will always be much interested. As long as the public—and I am sorry to say, medical men and others who ought to know better— cannot distinguish between the genuine and the false, between the hypnotic condition and the gross, and in many instances extremely gross imitations of it, "world renowned mesmerists," and "only living mesmerists," .will deluge town and country with their brazen lies,, and the public platform with their still more unblushing audacities.

Some of the most interesting and instructive entertainments I know of have been mesmeric in character. I do not think any other class of entertainment can be made so enjoyable or so innocent in character.

If the mesmerist is a physiognomist or phrenologist he will be able to tell what are the salient points in character which distinguish each subject, one subject from another. He will proceed accordingly, and endeavour to excite or exalt such faculties (by manipulation or suggestion, or both), which he desires to bring into plays. This he will accomplish much more successfully than an operator—however good a mesmerist—who cannot with equal faculty read character. For public entertainments, as well as in every other sphere of abour, the keen reader of character—all else being-equal—has the advantage over all others. What is true of the greater, cannot be false of the less. Therefore, the mesmerist in this respect is no exception to the rule.

To give a public entertainment it is a *sine qua non* that, for any hope of success in that direction,, the operator has had considerable practice in private, therefore, he is at home in his work, knows what he is about, what he has to do, and the difficulties with which he has to contend. That he has recognised, and is prepared to successfully overturn, the difficulties which may arise from the capricious fancies of his audience, and such difficulties as may arise from having few, none, or very subjects. He may be nervous and anxious; his audience may be small in numbers, ignorant or sceptical but be this as they may, he must have *perfect control over himself,* and ability to have *full* control over his audience. If he is not able either to control or entertain his audience, all his hope for success as an exhibitor or entertainer will be seriously shaken by failure. For confidence begets confidence, and success.

To succeed, he must not only be a good mesmerist, possess the utmost faith in his own powers, but he must be a usually .wide-awake person, adding to firmness, will resolution, ready fact, and keenness of observation, and thereby have complete command of his audience, as well as his subjects. He will often require to avert disaster, and either minimise failures, or turn them into undoubtable success. Occasionally some very clever people may come upon the platform, assume to be mesmerised, and up to a certain stage appear to do their part well, at the same time, when opportunity occurs, they make cabalistic signs with their thumb, fingers, and nose behind the operator's back to their confederates in the audience. The majority of audiences being composed of persons who come more for fun and amusement than instruction they are ready in consequence to enter into the spirit of the thing, which, if successful, may amuse, the audience but it means ruin to the entertainer. He must detect the fraud, and be ready to seize, a good moment to expose the humbug, and completely turn the ridicule upon him. By a clever movement the mesmerist will gratify his audience, secure their confidence, and continue to amuse them, and what is very important, with profitable results.

I remember in the city of Edinburgh a brilliant audience of nearly 2000 persons, in Newsome's Circus. Nicholson Street, was assembled to witness one of my mesmeric demonstrations. There was, however, a turbulent element present. Mesmerism, or Hypnotism, not being so fashionable then as now, a good number of medical men were present, as well as some three hundred and fifty of four hundred students. Some fun was anticipated by them. It was the "dominant idea," of the students, and, of course, would soon be expressed, scientifically in the "expectant." What a wonderful thing science is, what a disabuser of charms and fancies—what profundity of thought, what paucity of heart, and total annihilation of soul, characterise science in certain quarters. Well these young students had not yet attained to the full height of intellectual cramming; of heart and soul, doubtless they had plenty. However, in the present instance, such possessions were overshadowed by the fact that they had just had a rectoral election, and, for a day or two, they intended to make "Rome howl." Raids were organised upon various places of amusement. Mine was not to escape. The local people had made the necessary precautions. The students, baffled at the theatres and concerts, made a grand rush for Nicholson Street. Crowding through the entrances they soon filled up the gallery and what few vacant places that were to be found elsewhere. For a short time the tumult baffled description. The students shouted, whistled, spat peas through tin tubes, threw bags of flour on the unoffending people in the pit and reserved seats. Women screamed, and men muttered cures both loud and deep. Order of decorum there was none, save upon the platform. There my poor subjects were posed in various attitudes, with every expression of feature, from grave to gay, from lively to severe, utterly oblivious of what was taking place about them. The slightest timidity on my part would soon be communicated to them (some twenty in number, four of whom were my own sensitives, the balance were taken from the audience in the ordinary way). That was to be avoided. The slightest show of timidity would be a signal to the unfeathered bipeds—embryo medicos and divines—to be as heartless and as daring as possible. I also feared a collision between the audience and the students — the former were so indignant with the conduct of the latter. Amid the din and excitement, to reduce to order such chaos seemed to be a hopeless task. Nerved by the thought of my sensitives, and the financial consequences, I determined to make the effort. All this time my pianist was "playing like mad," thumping order cut of discord, in a vain endeavour to drown the noise by his music. I signalled to him to let the poor piano alone, and give his arms and fingers a rest. I walked up and down the platform as if about to do *something*— a habit which I had when I wished particularly to arrest the attention of an audience—and then suddenly faced the audience, and lifted my right hand and stood still. The major portion of the audience looked toward the platform. "Rule Britannia" and "Old John Brown" of the students were now reduced to fitful gusts. The element of curiosity had now slightly got ahead of "dominant idea of having a good night's fun. "What's he going to do now? became the undercurrent idea, I trusted to the innate love of fair play which is the characteristic of every Briton, although just now overshadowed by the horseplay peculiar to students at rectorial elections. I made several pantomimic motions indicating a desire for a "word." Taking advantage of a lull, secured by these efforts, I said—"Ladies and gentlemen, and particularly my young friends of the Edinburgh University who have just arrived, if you will permit me, I will tell you of a little incident which occurred a short time ago." (Slight booing and shouts of "go-ahead" and "wire in," from my cultured young friends, but general attention from the whole audience.) "A gentleman was out with a few friends; and his hounds hunting one day near Rathmines. They had succeeded in ousting an old fox; getting him into the open, they were soon after him with full cry. The hounds had out run the riders considerably. The fox was getting pretty tired of this sort of thing. He didn't think it was altogether right, to put it mildly, for *so many* to be *down on one*. So the fox stopped short too. The fox addressed the hounds cousteously, between puffs thus—'Gentlemen, what are you after?' 'We are out for a day's fun' said the puppy who led the hounds. 'Well, then, gentlemen,' said the fox, "It may be fun to you, but it is death to me." I tell the Aesopian story badly, but the effect was magical The people applauded, and the students sang, "For he's a jolly good fellow," and gave me no more trouble that evening or during my stay.

I turned my apparent defeat that night into a victory by a little coolness and tact. I asked the students and the audience to appoint a committee of six gentlemen—three medical and three nonmedical—to represent them on the platform, and keenly watch the experiments. This was done. At the close, the committee reported entired satisfaction with all that they had seen. They critically examined the subjects, and were perfectly satisfied with the genuineness of the phenomena which occurred through them. They also complimented me in no stinted manner; and no wonder. The opposition I met with that night and the determination to bring the whole to a happy issue, seemed to arouse in me all my energies, for it was certainly one of most complete exhibitions of mesmeric power I ever gave.

These experiments, out of many, Will serve as an illustration of what took place. In the first—with a Glasgow sensitive—I exhibited my complete control over the arterial circulation. Thus, while the subject stood placidly between two medical men, each holding a wrist and carefully taking the pulse indications, etc., I accelerated or retarded the action of the heart at will. Strange as this may appear, stranger must follow. I caused the pulse to reach 120 or 130 per minute on the right arm, and it beat less than 50 per minute on the left, and vice-versa. This can be explained on two grounds: either the subject was mesmerised by me, and the phenomena, as described, did occur (as testified to by these medical men at the time), or the medical men themselves were mesmerised by me, and, under my guidance, *hypnotically declared what was false to be true.* I might add that the subject was in a deep unconscious sleep; the medical men were apparently wideawake. The common-sense conclusion would be that the subject was mesmerised and not they; and that they, being wide awake and in the full possession of their senses, had testified to what they had seen. This experiment has been frequently repeated.

The second experiment was somewhat similar in character to the above. The medical gentlemen on the committee asked my permission to test the insensibility of the subjects. It was proposed to place a hot spirit-tube suddenly to different muscles to see if they flexed under the test, and thereby indicate the presence of nervous sensitiveness or consciousness. I made no objection to this. There was some difficulty in getting a spirit test-tube, so, to prevent unnecessary waiting, a gentleman lent a gold scarf-pin, and a lady her brooch, to the committee. I made the subject's arm rigid in a horizontal position. One of the medical committee men, feeling the carpus of the hand carefully, took the scarf-pin, and put it through the hand, about the centre, from back to front. He also placed the gold pin of the brooch through the sensitive's cheek, the brooch itself hanging on the outside, the poor fellow laughing and chatting as if nothing had happened. Neither by movement nor sign did he show he experienced any pain, or that he was the least conscious of what had taken place. When the audience, or rather their committee, were satisfied of this, I took the scarf-pin out of the hand and the brooch out of the cheek. *No blood flowed from the cicatrix.* Imagination, suggestion, are capable of doing strange things. The late and esteemed Dr. Carpenter claims much for the "dominant idea and expectancy." Can they account for the foregoing experiments?

Again, I either was instrumental in producing the extraordinary effect—phenomenon if you will — in the case by mesmerising the subject, or it was brought about by a much more extraordinary effort on my part, *i.e.*, I had mesmerised the committee and my audience, self-deception and fraud being out of the question. The common-sense view of the case is: I had such control over the sensitive that I stopped the flow of his blood, which, in ordinal circumstances, would have taken place. The committee, being satisfied with the result, testified to the fact.

The third experiment was not a pleasant one, but to the committee was as convincing as were the others. The committee desired me to produce two results—the first without contact, and the next any way I pleased. The directions were written on paper that I should cause the subject to stand erect, slowly raise his arms holding them out horizontal to his shoulders, and then gradually open out his legs, as if standing astride of something. I placed the subject facing the audience, and standing several feet in rear of him, I made passes in the direction of the position I wanted him to take up. Slowly, but surely, the sensitive responded to my mental efforts and mesmeric passes, and took up the position as designed by the committee.

The next experiment was to produce a cataleptic fit, which could not be distinguished in any of its pathological features from a case such as a medical man would meet in the ordinary course of practice. This was done by irregular phreno-manipulation and suggestion. The spectacle produced by the subject is not likely to be soon forgotten by either the committee or the audience. The man suddenly upon the platform with the despairing shout peculiar to that disease. The veins of the neck and head became engorged, the lips from a healthy red became a deep blue-black. The spasmodic struggles of the body and the irregular action of the heart confirmed the processes of the disease. I watched the case narrowly, so as not to prolong the condition, and be ready to entirely de-mesmerise the sensitive and relieve him of all unpleasant results.[1] The committee were more than satisfied. Mesmerism came triumphant out of the ordeal; and what at first appeared a defeat, a hopeless disaster, was changed into a victory.

During the remainder of my stay in Edinburgh namely, three weeks, I met with every courtesy from the medical profession and from the students. I had no further trouble—in fact, large number turned out every evening to learn as well as to be entertained.

In bringing this chapter to a close, I have reason to believe that the public idea of the use and abuses of Mesmerism is an

---

[1] Unpleasant as this experiment appears to be it is not without its modicum of good—viz., the same methods adopted to stay its progress will arrest and finally cure cataleptic fits, etc.

extravagant one. The claims in its favour are as often imaginative as those which call for its denunciation.

The following extract from the *Glasgow News* is a fair example:—"Lecturing in Glasgow recently. Professor M'Kendrick admitted the existence of a mesmeric—or, to employ the more fashionable term, hypnotic—power, and pointed out that it might be legitimately and usefully employed by medical men; but he strongly objected to the public exhibitions of professional mesmerists, as calculated to lead to the infliction, in some instances, of serious and permanent injury upon the 'subjects' experimented with. A case in point is reported from the south of England,, where a young lady of 'large property' is said to have lost her reason through the influence brought to bear upon her by an itinerant French 'hypnotist.' After having been mesmerised by this man, 'she did not seem to regain her full senses, but raved all night, and for several days, of the dark-eyed Gaul' At last she disappeared, and at the end of three days was discovered by the aid of the mesmerist, whom she had followed to France. Her condition is now described as one of 'raving madness' and she has been placed in a lunatic asylum. It is only fair to say that in this instance the operator does not seem to have had evil designs of any kind, and of course, the poor girl's malady might have developed itself without his intervention; but Mesmerism appears to have been the exciting cause, and at all events, the terrible possibilities suggested by the case should lend force to Professor M'Kendrick's warning."

"The dark-eyed Gaul," in my opinion, was in no way responsible for the result. Her "raving madness" would have soon ceased to be had he had any influence over her. Ignorant itinerants may do much harm, and ladies of property must be protected, but how about pauper and other humble patients in our hospitals hypnotised by budding medicos? Should not something be done for them?

CHAPTER VIII. HOW TO GIVE AN ENTERTAINMENT—(Continued).

Mesmeric entertainments are seldom or ever conducted on purely mesmeric principles. All stage phenomena are the product of combined forces. Some subjects may be mesmeric sensitives, others are hypnotised, while the majority are placed under your control by (what I shall call, for want of a better name) Mesmeric-Psychology. Both Animal Magnetism and suggestion are here called into play by yourself—aye, and imitation, imagination, ideas, Md lost sight of which can be judiciously used. Taking for granted that you have a good idea of Mesmerism in theory and practice, you may proceed to give your entertainment. Hitherto you have mesmerised persons singly, but now you are to operate on the mass. To facilitate matters, leave nothing to chance. As you have mesmerised in private, have some of your sensitives in the audience. Such sensitives you will keep in reserve for special experiments—clairvoyants for clairvoyant experiments, your susceptible subjects for experiments of will such as described in a previous chapter, your thought-reading subjects for special phases. Don't use any of these for general experiments, where illusion and phantasy are created by your suggestions. For the latter experiments you can depend largely upon the *impressible subjects* secured from your audience. You can proceed somewhat in this fashion: —Commence your entertainment by making a telling speech (the shorter the better) upon the subject. Quote authorities whose -names will have some influence with your audience. Detail some of the cures performed, cases of *Clairvoyance* (if any) which have come under your notice, or any little incident in thought-reading—psychometry—which will tell effectively. You can point out the value of Mesmerism to medical men and dentists as a powerful and harmless anaesthesia, under which will tell effectively. You can point out the value of Mesmerism to medical men and dentists as a powerful. and harmless anesthesia, under which patients may have surgical operations performed upon them, or teeth extracted without the slightest pain, etc. Give some of your experiences. If you are in earnest; therefore thoroughly interested in your subject, you will soon personally impress your audience, and prepare them to assist you in giving your entertainment.

The next thing you do is to ask for volunteers — *ordinary people from the audience*—to come upon the platform. While doing so, *impress* upon those you ask *"you will see that they came to no harm— you will take every care of them if mesmerised."* Those whom you are not able to get under influence can go back to their seats again and enjoy the performance. With the exception of one, let all the rest of your previously made subjects remain in the audience. It is a good thing for some one to lead the way after you give your invitation. The next thing to do is to especially impress upon the audience to keep as quiet as possible. Direct your musician to play something soft and sweet—kindly music, with "a dim religious light" in it—and thus assist the effect you wish to make on your audience and subjects. These latter can rather be seated facing the audience or sitting sideways. But if you are not sure of yourself, and desire all the artificial aid you can get, seat your subjects with their backs to the audience, so as to have the light of the hall upon their backs, but upon your face and *eyes*. In a large audience, especially in England, a large number of persons will volunteer. When they are seated cast your eyes rapidly along your lines, and reject *all* you think you will have any trouble with; politely but firmly ask them to go down. If you are not a phrenologist trust to common sense indications. If a person on sitting down immediately crosses his legs, throws back his head, invite him to go down. These are the sure signs of self-conscious superiority—of "knowingness." Don't waste time with such people. Reject all persons smelling of drink or tobacco.

Regarding those selected, ask them to neither wish to be influenced nor desire not to be, but place themselves in your hands and to follow your directions as faithfully as possible. You can then use one of the following methods to *lessen their brain activity, arrest attention, and secure control over them.* Give all your directions in a firm, resolute, distinct but natural voice; tell each person upon the platform "to place their left hand in the hollow of their right hand palm uppermost." Then see that this is done. Put a disc[2] in the centre of the uppermost hand of each person, then raise both hands of each within nine or twelve inches from their eyes. Tell them to look steadily at the object which you have placed there until you give them permission to do otherwise; you will then proceed to mesmerise your "own subject" in the ordinary way. His faking asleep will arouse the attention of your audience, and prepare the way for further effects. During all this time, your musician is playing as directed. It is a mere matter of form giving an old subject a disc to look at, as you can control them without, but their example has a silent and potent influence over the rest, and materially helps to bring about the desired result will the least fatigue to yourself.

You will now proceed to control your subjects. Commence with one or two persons (who have been influenced at some previous time. Take the disc, and put it in your pocket, and in a bag which you may have for the purpose. Tell the subject to "*close his eyes firmly or tightly*" over which you will make some rapid passes with *the intention of really closing them.* This done, place the thumb of your right hand upon the forehead of the subject, in

---

[2] The discs are made of zinc, about the size and thickness of a florin, having a copper rivet in the centre, the whole amalgamated with mercury. They have a slight voltaic influence and, are principally used for the above effects.

such a way as to lie across the root of the nose, just above the eyebrows. You will aid your intention with a *slight downward pressure*. With your left hand you will take the right hand of your subject in a natural and easy way. At the same time you bring your thumb pressure to bear on the forehead. You will press with the knuckle joint of the third finger of the right hand. The pressure must be simultaneous, with your thumb contact at the forehead. The magnetic or mesmeric circle will be complete. When you are making the contact, you will say in a firm and decided manner — *"Now—you—cannot—open —your—eyes."* You will invariably find that in the majority of persons whose eyes are not far apart, they cannot open their eyes (they may or may not be asleep). Proceed to another and another and do the same. Those whose eyes are closed, let them remain on the platform; send the rest down. My favourite method of getting control and influencing a great number of subjects at the same time (irrespective of the nature and character of the various types of phenomena likely to be presented by them is as follows: —When the requisite number of volunteers are secured, I direct each to settle down comfortably in their seats, to take and hold tightly the thumb of the left hand in the hollow of the right, dose their eyes,[3] and lean their heads back (generally against the back of their seats or against the wall). Standing at a distance of three or four feet from the subjects, I make a series of rapid downward passes — *at distans*—over all, commencing at the left end of the line, and working to the right, time occupied ranging from five to ten minutes. During which time all previously influenced subjects pass into the mesmeric state and are afterwards, if necessary, aroused into the somnambulistic or mesmeric psychological stage. The others who are not, apparently, effected by the general process, are treated personally to rapid downward passes over the eyes and down the

---

[3] This is done simply to withdraw the subjects' attention from their surroundings.

temples, then the *contact* is taken as described. In audiences varying from 200 to 2000 persons, I have no difficulty in getting all the subjects I want to give a successful entertainment I prefer the latter method, as clairvoyant, thought-reading, and good phreno-mesmeric sensitives were not spoiled as they would be by the *disc*-process.

Having obtained the requisite number of subjects, you will proceed with your experiments. Sometimes these may be general in character, in which all the subjects participate—illusion after illusion dexterously created in their minds by the combined influences of phreno-manipulation and suggestion. Such an experiment as the following is interesting; — Lead all your subjects into a garden (an imaginary one). Let them behold its beauties, enjoy its fruits, and gather its flowers. Give them all freedom of action and speech therein. Some will manifest greed and selfishness; others will be generous courteous, and kindly to a fault; some will eat greedily and see little of the picturesque in their surroundings. To others it will be a veritable garden of delight—the tint of the flower, the combination of foliage, there, the fore-ground here, the back-ground there, the blending lights and shades, and the perspective, the *tout ensemble* is to them a thing of beauty and a joy for ever. All according to their temperament and character, walk through and enjoy the living dream — for dream it is and nothing more. Discover a cluster of bees warming in some corner of the garden. Let me one, thoughtlessly or greedily searching for fruit, disturb the bees. The change of scene is magical. Some will desperately fight the bees; others will manifest rage; some will sit down and try to cover themselves from attack while others will cry like children. In all this, you give the natural faculties of each their action as in dream. Again find a little grave, read the pathetic story which the epitaph unfolds, and by gradual transition lead your whole party into a cemetery or necropolis (as in dreaming, your subject will pass

112

from one stage to another without question). Here, again, you let the faculties have full play. One will sit and reflect on boy-hood's days, and the companionship of friends now gone; another win plant a rose bush by the grave of a friend— a little brother or child; a thoughtless youth will shed abundant tears, real tears, by the grave of his mother —upon being judiciously questioned, will perhaps admit that "he has been rather thoughtless and wayward," "has not been living just as his mother would like him to do, and now he is truly sorry for it," and may promise amendment. (I have succeeded in getting many subjects to give up tobacco and drink, and forego other habits by promises give me in this state, which they afterwards faithfully adhered to in their waking state. You can continue this pleasing experiment, with its various manifestations in the different subjects, for some little time. Make your musician play some lively dance music, and in a short time the crying, sobered, and distressed ones will forget all about the graveyard and its associations, and commence with hearty energy to trip the light fantastic toe in the gay exuberance of the merry dance. As soon as you observe them all in interesting or statuesque attitudes *fix* them suddenly therein, by a sharp noise (such as the clapping of your hands together and the stamp of your foot on the platform would make, the music suddenly ceasing at the same time). The effect is remarkable. Your audience will follow each change suggested with interest, and greet the final tableaux with hearty, unstinted applause. Some operators release or de-mesmerise their subjects after each experiment. This is unnecessary — a waste of time and energy, without compensating effect.

You may then take a subject and catalepse him, make his body, or any portion thereof, as rigid as a board. Take one of the foregoing subjects, de-mesmerise his legs and body by lateral and upward passes. Get him to stand erect in the centre of the platform. Make passes from the head down to the spine, and from the tophead down to the finger tips and to the heels. These passes being made with *the intention of making the subject rigid,* and of exhibiting your influence over the nerves of motion, etc. When this is done, stand behind him a little distance, and make passes towards him with the intention of pulling him back, and he will fall into your hands. Lay him down carefully on his back upon the ground. Release four of your statues, inform them that this poor fellow is very ill, or has been found drowned, etc., and let them act out their dreaming, for a few minutes, and the effect will be exceedingly interesting.

You may then suggest that the person (catalepsed subject) be taken to the police-station infirmary, or dead-house, as the case may be. Tie a white handkerchief around the subject's fore-head—to heighten effect, with two subjects to his shoulders, and the other two to his feet. Let them carry him shoulder high—(the musicians playing something funeral). They will now march with the dead man, followed (if you so direct) by all the other subjects, weeping and bemoaning the loss of their supposed friend.

As far as possible, concentrate the attention of all the subjects upon the apparently dead man. Let them lay his imaginary grave, and just as they are about to bury him, de-mesmerise his limbs, relax all his muscles, make him spring to his feet, and impress upon the others that he is a ghost risen from the grave, and a scene will take place which will baffle the pen of a ready writer. Some will jump the stage and secret themselves in different parts of the hall; others will hide themselves behind chairs and forms upon the platform; some crying others praying, all more or less frightened, etc. When this has been sufficiently prolonged your supposed dead man can be made suddenly to deliver a speech, or sing a song. —milk a cow, or something else; equally well contrasted with his former position, to the complete astonishment and mystification of your audience. The successful entertainer must be prepared to spring: a series of surprises on his audience.

With mesmeric psychological subjects although an amount of bodily energy and mental will-power are necessarily exerted in preparing them, the mental and physical exhaustion of giving an entertainment is after all more apparent than real. Kind friends and the majority of an audience will give you credit for great exertions and greater loss of vital energy and mental force, etc., than you really deserve. The most successful public mesmerists are naturally healthy men. Personally I don't believe either that they or myself were even more exhausted in giving a first-class entertainment than most other persons would be in giving a good and telling lecture, a night's reading, or sermon. These subjects when once under influence, are easily and readily dominated by the mesmerist's will and control. Even with those subjects who are conscious, and whose reason rebels by obvious facts from a suggested idea, the idea ultimately prevails, and the subjects will only see and think eventually as the mesmeriser may direct. The field of illusion is so extensive, for, as in phantasy and dreaming, it is interminable.

Under the influence of the operator, there is absolutely no end to the illusions which may be created in the subject's mind and acted upon 'without question. Fertility of resource and direction are requisites in an entertainer more than so-called extraordinary will-power (effort and exhaustion) to which success is often attributed. Most subjects can be awakened by wafting a handkerchief rapidly before the face, and throwing thereby a cold steam of air into the lungs, and thus increase the circulation and the blood supply to the brain, or by striking the subject upon the shoulder a sharp blow with the open hand, and shouting, "Awake, Awake!" Before leaving the platform all subjects should be thoroughly de-mesmerised. During the entertainment, it is sometimes necessary to remove one impression before creating another, such as the effect of sudden joy, fear or dread—frights and surprises. This can be readily done by upward passes, two or three, or by exclaiming, loudly and decidedly. "Right, right" followed by inquiring *in sotto* voice, "All right." As soon as the subject gets over his surprise, he will smile and look "all right."

It is here, I admit, that *suggestion* has a large field for exercise. Braid, Charcot, Carpenter, and others, however, err in supposing—that all Mesmerism is the result of suggestion. A detailed list of experiments suitable for an entertainment would not serve any useful purpose here. It is a good plan, if you have good clairvoyant or thought-reading subjects to use them sparingly, the result will be more satisfactory. A very telling experiment, if a subject has a really bad tooth—which is not and can never be of any use to him, is to throw him asleep upon the platform and have some well-known local dentist to extract it. The extraction will be a painless one, and the experiment most interesting. Never allow subjects to eat and drink anything which can in any sense do them an injury, or allow abusive liberties to be taken with them under the pretence of proving that your entertainment is like Caesar's wife — above suspicion.

INTERESTING EXPERIMENTS IN
THE WAKING STATE.

If you wish to ascertain whether you have an influence over a person, ask him to stand, place his keels together, and put his hands down by his side. Stand behind such a person, place your hands upon his shoulders for a few minutes, then concentrate your *passes* down his spine to the small of his back. These passes are made as if charging the spine your influence. Having done so several times, place the tips of your fingers lightly upon the back, level with the lower part of the shoulder blades, and proceed to make drawing passes, with the intention of drawing the person to you. In a great number of cases you will succeed in doing so. All such persons can be mesmerised, or otherwise psychologically influenced. This is called Testing Susceptibility. Or place your hands upon the shoulders in such a way that your thumbs converge and point toward the spine, just between the shoulder blades, *will strongly* that he fall backwards, towards you. If he responds readily he will make a good psychological subject; tardily, a good mesmeric subject. If not influenced, it may be a question of time. Should he go from you, it is more than likely you cannot *influence* him at any time.

Or, let the person stand as before, ask him to place his hands, palms down, fair and square on the top of yours—yours being palms uppermost. Will that his hands, become fastened to yours, so that he cannot pull them away, try he ever so hard. The best plan is not to say what you intend to do until you are ready, then say quietly and firmly. *"Now you cannot take your hands away."* The struggling and grimaces which follow will afford plenty of innocent mirthfulness to all concerned. This is called Fascination.

Or, take his right hand and place it on top of your left hand, and make a number of passes down his arm and over his hand, with the intention of fastening his hand to yours. Continue this for a little time, and then make passes (with your right hand) down in front of his body to his knees, as if charging his body and less with your influence; then, make drawing passes at the knees with the intention of causing him to kneel. In a short time he will go down unresistingly upon his knees much to his astonishment; and the amusement of others present, and perhaps of himself.

Or, let him sit upon a chair and cross one leg over the other. Right or left leg—it is immaterial. Make passes over the uppermost leg for a little, as if charging, and then proceed to make drawing passes surely the foot will rise toward you with every pass, in spite of all efforts made to the contrary. Once in position, inform the subject that he cannot put his leg down. As you have succeeded in lifting the foot up, you may be sure he will not be able to put it down without your permission. When you wish him to put it down, pat the leg briskly on the outside from the foot up to the thigh, then say decidedly, "*Now* you can put it down." The muscles being relaxed, he will be able to do so with ease. There are a great variety of similar experiments which may be carried out upon persons when wide awake all the time, which can do no harm, and give much amusement. Aye, and something more—far more valuable than the foregoing. Where you possess such control, your *influence* power, and sympathy over disease will be truly marked. You win begin to understand, from such apparently trivial results, *that the great value of Mesmermn lies in its power to alleviate the sufferings of humanity.* The curative is everything. The foregoing experiments are suitable either for drawing-room or platform.

The class of experiments which always gave most satisfaction to me are those which are produced by will and by manipulation. The most successful are those known as phreno-mesmeric— referred to elsewhere—and were largely adopted by myself in public entertainments with the most gratifying an astonishing results. The majority public mesmerists, having more faith in themselves than any real knowledge of the subject, and being very distant copies of Grimes, Darling, and Stone—the American "biologists"—make a great fuss upon the stage, shout, stamp and stare at their subjects, and actually tell them what to do. Of course, the public laugh and enjoy to the full the incongruities and mirth-provoking antics of the conscious and semi-conscious victims of suggestion under the influence of such operators. With the phreno-mesmerist there is no noise. When his introductory speech is finished, he has but little to say for the rest of the evening—

producing all the desired effects by a *touch* here and *tip* there, on the head and face of his subjects. The earnest, tearful prayer—immoderate laughter — passionate weeping—amorous dalliances—absurd and impossible situations, are gracefully and naturally taken up and carefully enacted (as easily as if the persons operated upon had been under careful training for years), as the mesmeriser now excites an organ or a facial muscle by his *magnetic* touch.

With mesmeric sensitives, avoid all haste and suggestion. In a sense, take what comes—and you will have in due time the best results, clairvoyance and what not.

With phreno-mesmeric sensitives also avoid haste and suggestion as far as the latter can be eliminated from your experiments. The phenomena induced are sometimes traceable to the excitement of the cerebral organs by touch and sometimes to your will, and in some instances to both. Suggestion is possible when the sensitive understands the location of the faculties.

With mesmeric-psychological subjects, who form the great majority of all platform assistants, force results—*make what suggestions you please*. Ever bear in mind, while entertainment and entertaining have their uses, they are not the end all and be all of Mesmerism. Let your suggestions be wholesome, happy, healthy, and beneficial, elevating character always. Never descend to practical jokes, or to aught hurtful or unpleasant, simply to gratify your own vanity, sense of the ridiculous, or to amuse others, at the expense of your subject's health and happiness.

There is something inexpressibly funny in seeing a sedate old man forget his sedateness, and make passionate avowals of affection to a supposed young lady (who is another man dressed up in a poke-bonnet and shawl), or becoming the end man for a troupe of Christy Minstrels; personating some actor, or delivering a temperance address; feeding a bundle -of clothes or a handkerchief for a baby, using a hat for the pannada and a walking-stick for a spoon. All this may be produced by *suggestion*—with a thousand variations; but what then, if this is all. It would be better that there was no such thing as Mesmerism. Fortunately this is not all, as already shown in the preceding pages. While mesmeric entertainments amuse, they may be used successfully to draw attention to the more special and scientific aspects of this subject.

CHAPTER IX PHRENO-MESMERISM.

PROFESSOR CHARCOT has unexpectedly brought us back to the days of Animal Magnetism. He has effected some curious experiments on hysteron-epileptic patients in the Salpetriere Hospital, producing catalepsy and somnambulism at will. The subject placed for a few seconds or minutes before the full blaze of an electric light, becomes fascinated. The anaesthetic state is complete, for he can be pinched, etc., without exhibiting pain. The members retain whatever attitude is given them. The patient has become cataleptic. In vain you speak or question him. Place him in a tragic posture, the physiognomy becomes severe, and the eyebrows contract. Bring the hands together as in prayer, the visage softens and the features become supplicating. Cut off the light, the patient drops into a somnambulistic state he falls backward, the eyelids dose, and if the skin be rubbed, the part will contract as if under the influence of electricity. Call the patient, he will rise up and walk towards you. Tell him to kneel and he win kneel; to write and he will write; to sew, and he will, mechanically, like a slave, the eyes being firmly dosed. Sometimes the answers given are more intelligible than when the patient is wide awake, so much is the intelligence excited. Blow in his face and the subject instantly awakens, after a slight throat spasm and some froth on the lips, but utterly ignorant of what has occurred. The experiment can be repeated at will. Music—strong bell-ringing—can produce this anaesthetic condition as well as the lights referred to; hence, the action of sound is identical with that of light. Steadily looking into the eyes will also produce the lethargic state. But this is treading after Mesmer." [*Translated*]

This is an interesting part of the subject. Unfortunately the majority of the public are not much acquainted with the Mental Science, as founded upon Phrenology—Phrenology with many is a vulgar something about "bumps." They believe in physiognomy—*i.e.*, the temperament, quality of organisation, disposition, and tendency of character as revealed in the face. Of the physiognomy of the head—Phrenology—however, they know nothing. They understand the clock dial, the hands thereon, and the time indicated there and by them; but of the nature and power of the machinery behind the dial, they are ignorant. So there are too many who care little for the cerebral machinery, its form, size, quality, and power—by which the mind animates the face indicating thereon the morning, the mid-day, and the twilight of the human soul in Time. To appreciate Phreno-Mesmerism, some knowledge of Phrenology is requisite. The successful mesmerist must either be a keen physiognomist or a good phrenologist. In the latter case, his psychological experiments will be the most satisfactory and fascinating. Sensitives in the deep mesmeric sleep, and who are conscious of your thoughts, or otherwise in full sympathy or *en rapport* with yourself, are not subjects for phreno-mesmeric experiments. The experiments with them, at least, would not be conclusive. In the somnambulistic state when the subject is deprived of consciousness, and is so far rendered oblivious as not to remember what has occurred during sleep unless *impressed* to remember —in this state the cerebral organs of the mental faculties resemble a piano—when excited by mesmeric influence they give forth manifestations in accordance with Phrenology, and the experiments are most effective and conclusive. The phenomena are not the result of *suggestion*, accident or imagination. In the majority of cases the sensitives, as one of the general public, can have no possible knowledge of Phrenology.

It is not possible for the experimentalist to be successful in this particular department without a thorough knowledge of Mesmerism on the one hand, and Phrenology on the other. The frequent failures which are sure to accompany a "little knowledge" have led many experiments to declare that phreno-mesmeric phenomena are either exceedingly fugitive in character, or where determined, are due to coincidence, accident, imagination, etc. I shall neither explain nor defend Phrenology here, but content myself with pointing out (that predicated on temperament) some persons are more susceptible to mesmeric influence than others. Of these, even in the sleep (and based on the same physiological conditions of organisation), some are more dull, or less susceptible than others. Persons of the mental and mental-vital temperament are more sprightly and vivacious, respond more readily to influence, than those of more stolid and less impressive natures. The former will respond to the lightest touch. In some cases, contact is not even necessary. The latter require decided and continuous pressure before the cerebral more stolid and less impressive natures. The former organs respond. Again, the first mentioned are, perhaps, the most difficult subjects to reduce to sleep; but when fully under influence, they make the best possible subjects for all forms of mental or psychological phenomena—thought-reading, thought-transference, psychometry, and phreno-mesmerism, etc. In the mesmeric state, under the peculiar nervous conditions induced by it, the whole brain, especially that of animal life and sense, is in a dormant or benumbed state. The somnambulistic state is often brought about by partial de-mesmerisation, as in semi-waking and sleeping dreams. By this phreno-mesmeric process, certain organs are stimulated into activity—and a direction, a positive direction under the control of the mesmerist, given to the thoughts and actions of the sensitive. Some doubt the possibility of such operations, yet admit the probability of the foregoing experiments of Charcot, based on automatic inhibition,—mechanical automatic suggestion, if you will. The greater includes the less, phreno-mesmeric processes, antedate Charcot's suggestions, and are superior to them. The former produce results, when the latter inevitably falls. By the former, we have direct communication with the brain—the organ of the mind; by the latter, mechanical and inhibitory suggestions are indirectly conveyed to the brain, and automatically responded to. By the former we have a living sensitive being, in a certain state of mental exaltation, giving forth some perfect manifestations of such psychological state.

In the latter, you have a degraded tool, a helpless piece of organic machinery— a marionette, "pull the strings and the figure moves."

The phreno-mesmeric process is as follows: — Put your subject in a deep unconscious sleep. As you can de-mesmerise or stimulate a leg or arm into activity, recognise the fact—the same can be accomplished with the brain, consciousness can be restored partially or wholly. The mind, directed by the influence of the operator, determinedly applied to the organ of the faculty desired to be aroused, by touching the organ or organs which you desire to affect, almost immediately the arterial blood is attracted and propelled with greater force through that portion of the brain; the faculty, or faculties, become exalted, or inspired. Excite "Imitation," and "Language." Foreign languages will be repeated verbatim, without hesitation or flaw, the subject having no knowledge of the language thus employed. Excite "Language," "Tune," and "Mirthfullness," the subject will probably sing some amusing and witty song. Excite "Language," "Veneration," and "Spirituality," the face of the sensitive will be reverent, devotional, and flooded with hallowed light; his invocations to the Deity will be most impressive and devout. Excite "Destructiveness" and energy, activity, possibly passion and temper, will be manifested. "Acquisitiveness" will indicate a desire to have; while "Benevolence" a desire to give. The special direction of either will depend upon what other organs are excited in unison therewith.

To allay the cerebral excitement, blow steadily on the organ or organs affected.

Drs. Elliotson, Braid, Spencer T. Hall, Mr. Atkinson, W. Jackson, Sergeant Cox, and others, paid considerable attention to this branch of experiments. Dr. Spencer Hall is naturally the authority whose experiments were to me the most interesting. Many of these were carried out upon persons in the waking as well as in the sleeping condition.

Two or three instances will suffice to illustrate this part of the subject. During some public experiments given by the writer in the Queen's Hall, Bold Street, Liverpool, about eleven years ago, one of the subjects kept time to the music by a lateral movement of his head. Desirous of testing the effect, I instructed the musicians to make a noise—in discordant musical notes, made in rapid succession, without rhythmic connection. The subject ceased to move his head, shuddered, and looked painfully distressed. On asking what was the matter, he replied he had a severe pain in his head, pointing at the same time to the organ of "Tune." On directing the musicians to play the "Blue Danube" waltz, the lateral movement of the subject's head commenced again. The discordant experiment was tried once more, with similar but intensified results. I was now quite satisfied. I blew upon the organ, and eventually carefully de-mesmerised the subject, and released him from all further influence that evening, reserving him afterwards—according to my usual practice—for phreno-mesmeric experiments only.

In every instance the natural language of each faculty was perfectly, and most beautifully manifested under influence; also in a way, I believe, not possible to the sensitive in his waking state. Captain John James, in writing on the matter, says: —"An uneducated man for instance, may, for the first time in his life be thrown into the mesmeric sleep-waking state, and the operator, by touching, and sometimes even by merely pointing at, the organ— say of 'benevolence'—may cause the sensitive to exhibit mortal signs of that particular sentiment, so that he may appear to fancy of dream that he sees before him some pitiable object, which at once awakens his interest and compassion. If "combativeness" be touched he will immediately show symptoms of anger, fancy he is quarrelling with someone, evince a desire to fight, and may even strike his mesmeriser; *fan* or *blow* over the excited organ, or touch 'benevolence,' and his anger immediately subsides. Should 'combativeness' and 'destructiveness' be very small, the excitement of the organ will often lead him to imagine that some one is trying to quarrel with him; neither the expression of his countenance nor his actions betraying any feeling of anger."

He further adds: —"The most interesting results in these experiments take place when two or more of the organs are simultaneously excited, when you will probably observe such beautiful combinations of graceful attitudes and facial expression, as would be well worthy the observation and study of a first-rate actor."

It frequently happens that a successful mesmerist may have no knowledge of Phrenology. As such he would fail in these experiments. It also happens that many very able phrenologists are not mesmerists, or, being mesmerists/have neither time nor disposition to use their powers, so that the foregoing class of experiments have fallen very much into disuse.

Personally, I am satisfied that in the majority of cases, the *mesmeric touch* will convey, adequate *stimuli*, in some way to the localised nerve-centres of the brain, and is the true cause of the phenomena, the response in all cases depending upon temperamental condition and brain-development of the subject.

There are some cases where the will of the operator is communicated to the subject by the means of the *touch* and it may be possible that both touch and the will, combined may affect the sensitive; but seldom is the result produced by will alone.

I have successfully affected patients through a third person, my medium for operating, and the person operated on, being equally ignorant of the phrenological locality of the faculties.

The subject deserves the fullest and most complete investigation. It is mentioned here in the hope that it may stimulate the study of Phrenology.

CHAPTER X. HOW TO MESMERISE ANIMALS.

ANIMALS are much more easily hypnotised than mesmerised. Domestic animals are affected more easily than others which do not so readily come within the natural controlling influence of man. A snake will fascinate a bird, a child and sometimes a man. To withstand the glare of a rattlesnake's eye with self-command is no easy matter. It has been, done. Men have been known to creep on hands and knees slowly and deliberately up to a rattlesnake, and just as it was about to spring and strike, seize it by the neck with the left hand, and cut off its head by a stroke of the bowie-knife in the right hand.

Tales of Eastern travel are full of incidents of snake-charmers, or tamers. The methods used are mesmeric in character. I have known persons who could control "beasts not bodies"—that is animals, but not human being, and others who had no influence over the former, but were very successful with the latter. This is a matter largely of temperament, natural aptitude, and association. Notwithstanding this, all may learn something about it. A reasonable amount of perseverance and practice will demonstrate whether you have a requisite gifts or not.

Certain persons evince great control over horses. They have certain secrets which they divulge, under special arrangements, to those who wish to learn their art. Sullivan and Rarey, the celebrated horse-tamers, were men who had special secrets. We have "Australian" "Hungarian," and "American" horse-trainers, who from time to time, appear before the British public and accomplish with success what ordinary trainers fail to do. Vicious horses, unbroken and wild colts, etc., are subdued in an hour or two by their influence. No doubt these men have a special knack. They have more than a knack—they have a *special process.*

Sullivan would walk into the stable of the most vicious and uncontrollable horse; in an hour after, he would lead the horse out, and do anything with him he pleased—having in that hour's time gained perfect control over the animal. Rarey performed similar feats. Neither of these men allowed anyone to enter the stable with them. The Arab, from close association, kindness, and due consideration for his steed, and from a knowledge of its nature and requirements, obtains perfect control over it. It is docile and obedient—the slightest sign of movement made by his master, is at once taken up and acted upon. The control and influence of the horse tamer is not like that of the Arab, a question of life association, of years, or months; but of one short hour. It must be a special power or gift possessed and used by the latter, which is not the case with the former, or even the majority of persons who have specially to do with horses, or else the high fees paid for the services of such men would not be given if what they are able to do could, even in a fair way be accomplished by others. The power exercised is magnetic or mesmeric in character. Years of constant use and concentration have intensified the gift and the power to use it. If the fear of man or beast, snake or bird, is experienced or left by the mesmerist, it is idle to attempt to mesmerise. To mesmerise a horse, or obtain control over him, there must be neither fear nor rashness possessed by the operator. He is also more likely to be successful if he possesses a sufficient knowledge of horses—temperament and disposition—to approach them in a natural and easy way. Taking, then, the foregoing for granted the following is the most effective way to control a vicious horse, and get him completely under your influence. Enter the stable, bar the door, walk rapidly and decidedly up to the horse in the stall, take the halter off his neck (keep close to his head, he can rear and snap as much as he likes), seize him by the forelock with the right hand and by the nostrils with the thumb and forefinger of the left hand, closing them upon the septum or cartilage dividing the nostrils with a tight grip, as a ring is fastened on a bull's nose. Make sure of your hold. Draw the horse's head down, and *blow strongly steadily into his ear* for about five minutes. He will soon cease to plunge and snap, and will stand trembling from head to feet. Give him two or three gentle pats on the shoulder, speak firmly and calmly as if to a human being, and then make passes from between the ears to as far down the back as you can reach without letting go his nose with your left hand. Should be attempt to break from you, plunge-rear, or kick, grasp tightly with your right hand, his forelock, or better still, his ear, draw his head down again and repeat the above. The moment he is quiet again, resume the passes and the patting. Passes can be made afterward from the top of the head down to the nostrils. The horse may then be directed to do certain things —to "back," "fee up," or "whoa," within the limits of the stable or stall. The breathing process and the passes to be repeated the moment he is refractory, until submission and obedience to your orders are assured. You then can lead him out of the stable, and with the long reins and whip give him some work—ring exercise, walking, running, etc.,—till there is a visible perspiration on his coat. When this is done take him into your stable-yard again. Brush and rub him well down. Let him cool a little. Repeat the foregoing for one hour a day for a week, and you will have no trouble with him afterward. A prolongation of the passes will put him asleep.

Dogs, cats, rabbits, are easily mesmerised. In fact, all animals frequently patted and rubbed with the hand from the head down the back, or over the spine, become very tractable and attacked to those who do so. Passes steadily over the eyes, and down to the nose, produce sleep. When the animal trembles, or becomes fidgety it is a good sign; continue the passes—operate as you would on a human being with *intention*. It is best not to close the animal's eyes with your fingers, but continue short local passes until the eyes close of their own accord, or the pupils become dilated.

When the animal is mesmerised, you can roll it about, pass a light before its eyes, and it will be insensible to such action. Call it by name, and, unless catalepsed, it will demurely follow you. The eye is a powerful agent in mesmerising animals as well as man. Dogs will succumb to the eye after they have resisted all passes and *effort* to mesmerise them in that way. To de-mesmerise an animal, take a pocket-handkerchief, waft it rapidly over it, call it by name, and it will soon "come to" all right.

Goats are easily mesmerised. Birds, pigeons, and canaries, and farm-yard fowl are readily influenced. For instance, interest the attention of a lively canary. Move your hand from right to left gently on a level with its head and eyes, at a distance of ten or twelve inches from the cage and gradually move nearer and nearer with shorter passes until, within an inch or two from the bird, when it will dose its eyes and fail asleep and off its perch. The larger brained the canary the more permanent will be his sleep, A clap of the hand, or sudden noise of any kind, will cause it to wake; whether he is awakened by yourself or by accident, always de-mesmerise — *i.e.*, by up and down passes, and blowing upon him.

Pigeons and poultry are most easily affected. The quickest action is hypnotic; the result, sleep. Take a game-cock; pick him up in a fighting mood; place him upon a table; make several passes with your forefinger ever his head and down his beak, he will soon be docile enough. To hypnotise him, tie his legs together with a piece of string, and place him on the floor or table before a line drawn with chalk, in a few minutes he will become quite passive. Untie the string, shove him about he is quite indifferent. Put his head under his wing, he will keep it there. Lay him on the floor in any position he will not attempt to move. To awake, use the handkerchief, and make a sudden noise.

To hypnotise a pigeon: put a small piece of white putty on the end of its beak, hold it steadily for a minute till its attention is arrested by the object; the eyes will converge, as in the human subject, and the pigeon will be hypnotised; it sleeps, or becomes rigid, but cannot be made to do any thing in this state. Pigeons, however, are readily trained.

Wild animals can be mesmerised. It is good practice for would be mesmerisers to visit the Zoological Gardens, or a good menagerie, and practice the art of arresting the attention of encaged beasts by gazing fixedly at them. This may not always be satisfactory, but it is good practice. Skate, or ray and other fish, are susceptible to the influence, but *cui bono*.

Much is permissible if the power of the operator is intensified and concentrated thereby and he is fitted to exercise his powers more effectually for the benefit of his fellows. To this end practice on animals, etc., has its value.

CONCLUDING REMARKS.

I think it is very right to say that in a brief work like this, I could only touch the borders of a great subject. The more subtle phenomena of Telepathy, clairvoyance, Thought-Reading. Thought-Transference, and Psychometry, indicative of soul or spirit in man, have, confessedly, only been glanced at. It has been esteemed wise, however, to make this beginning of the study of Mesmerism as practical and interesting as possible. To that end instructions have been given which are not to be found in more expensive publications. There are many useful and valuable books on Mesmerism not in circulation and only to be found in the British Museum, which unfortunately places them out of the reach of the reading public—(from some of these I have made extracts). What has been said in this brochure may lead to further inquiry, and to those who wish to take a more thorough interest in the subject of Mesmerism, I suggest they should read the works of Gregory, Heidenhain, Binet and Fere, Dods, Deleuze and Captain James, etc. However valuable reading may be, practical instruction at best can only be poorly conveyed by such means, and those who are really anxious to know "How to Mesmerise," should add to the information gleaned from books, the personal or voce directions of an experienced instructor or the writer.

THE END

www.ingramcontent.com/pod-product-compliance
Lightning Source LLC
Chambersburg PA
CBHW070033030426
42335CB00017B/2409